Cannabis The Cat
Goes to Washington

Written by
Jerry Frye

Illustrations by
Mike Motz

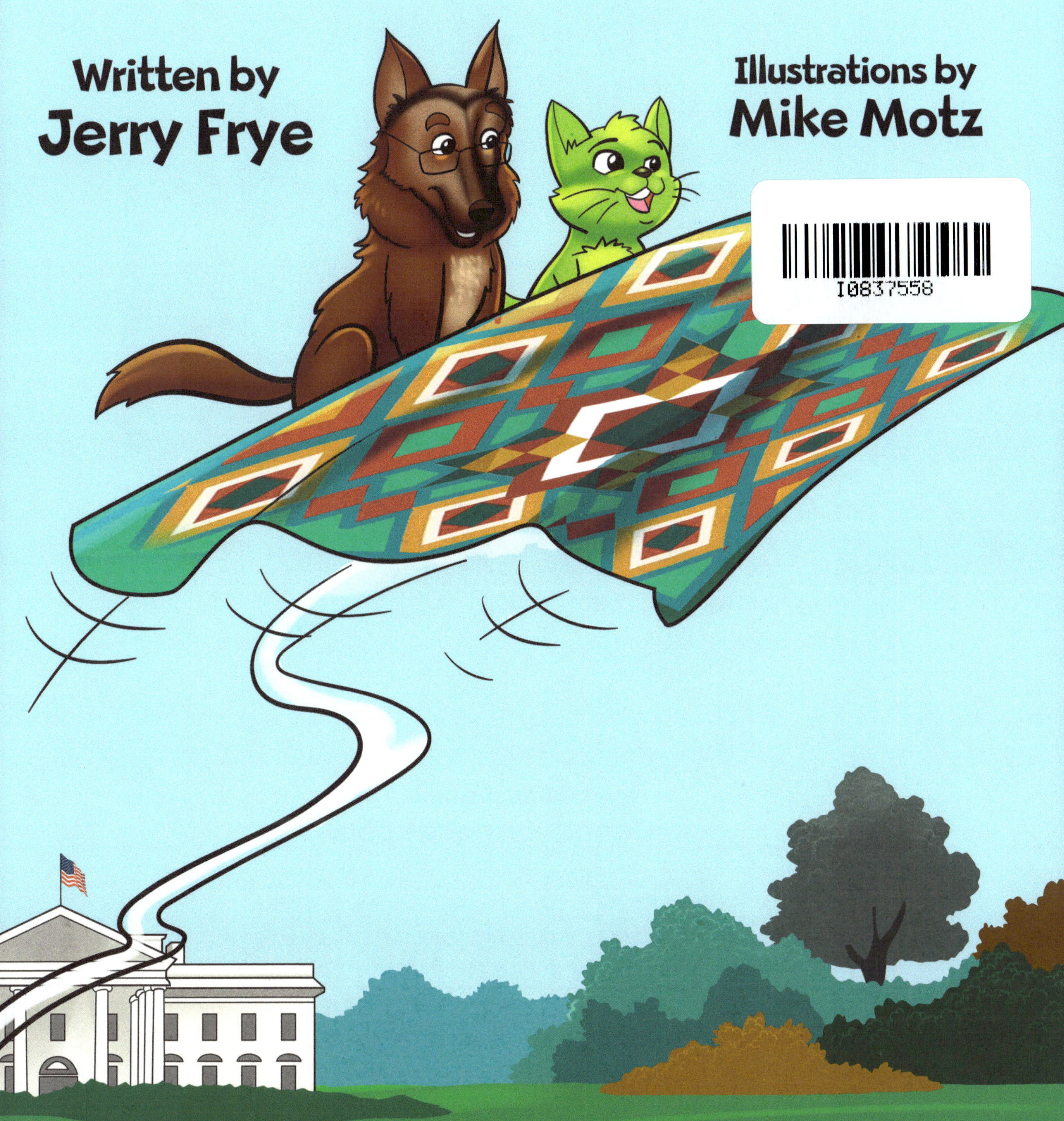

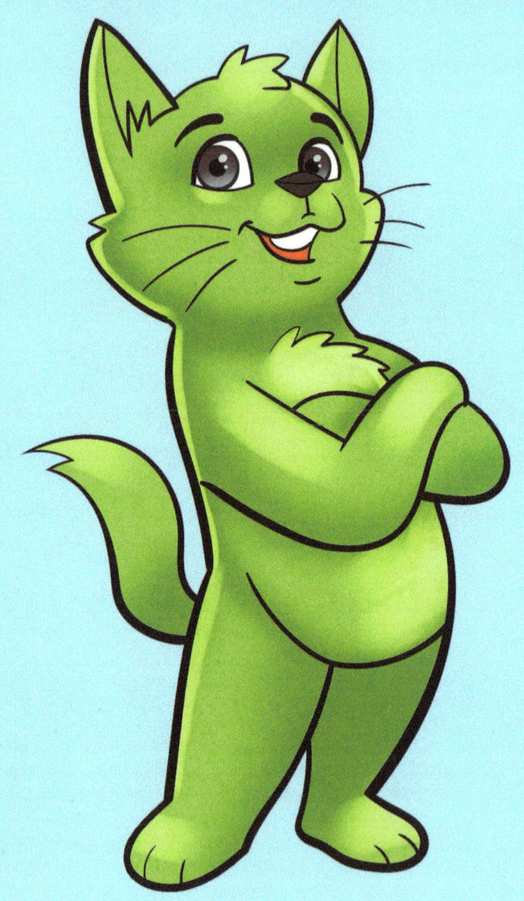

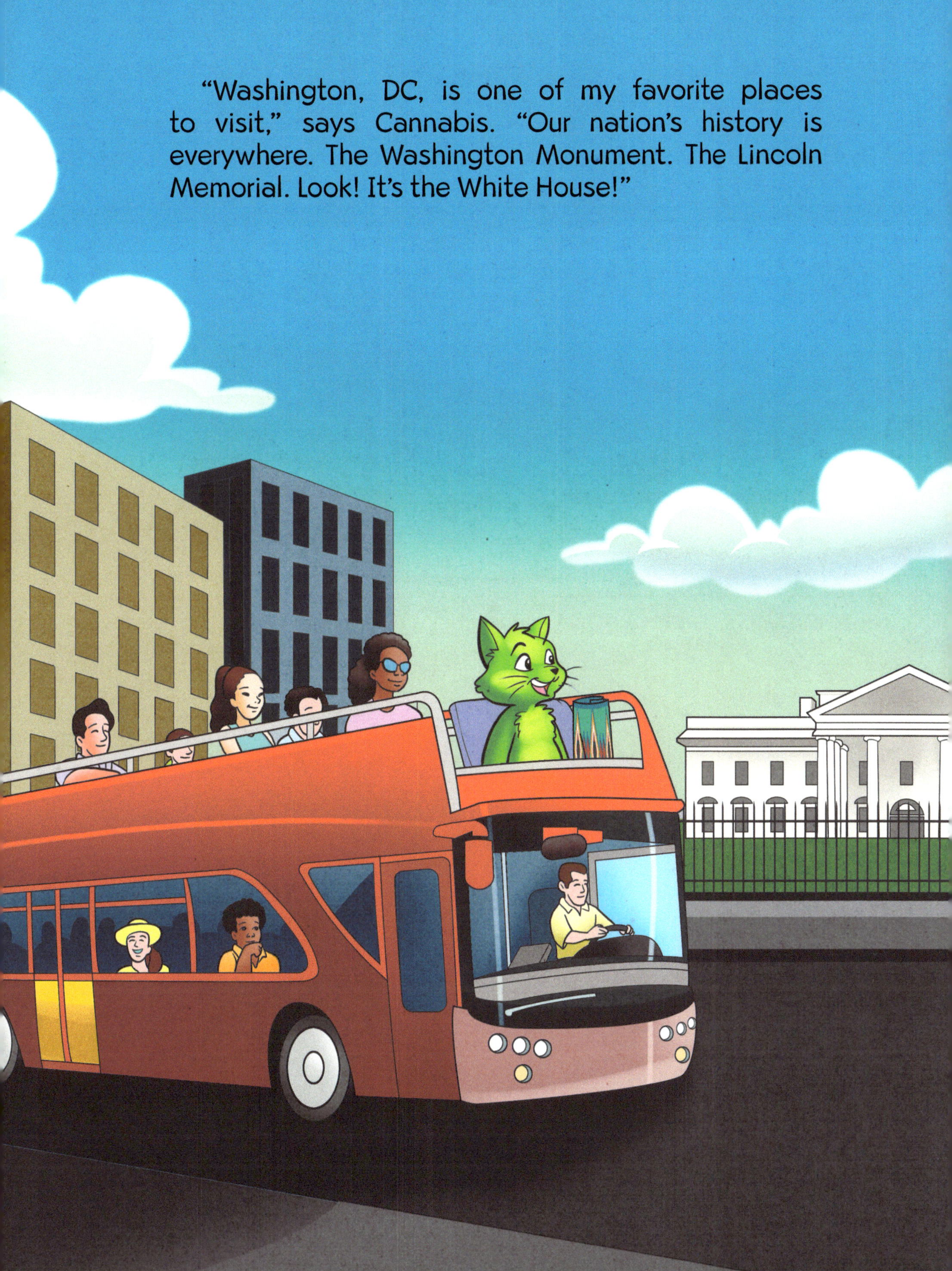
"Washington, DC, is one of my favorite places to visit," says Cannabis. "Our nation's history is everywhere. The Washington Monument. The Lincoln Memorial. Look! It's the White House!"

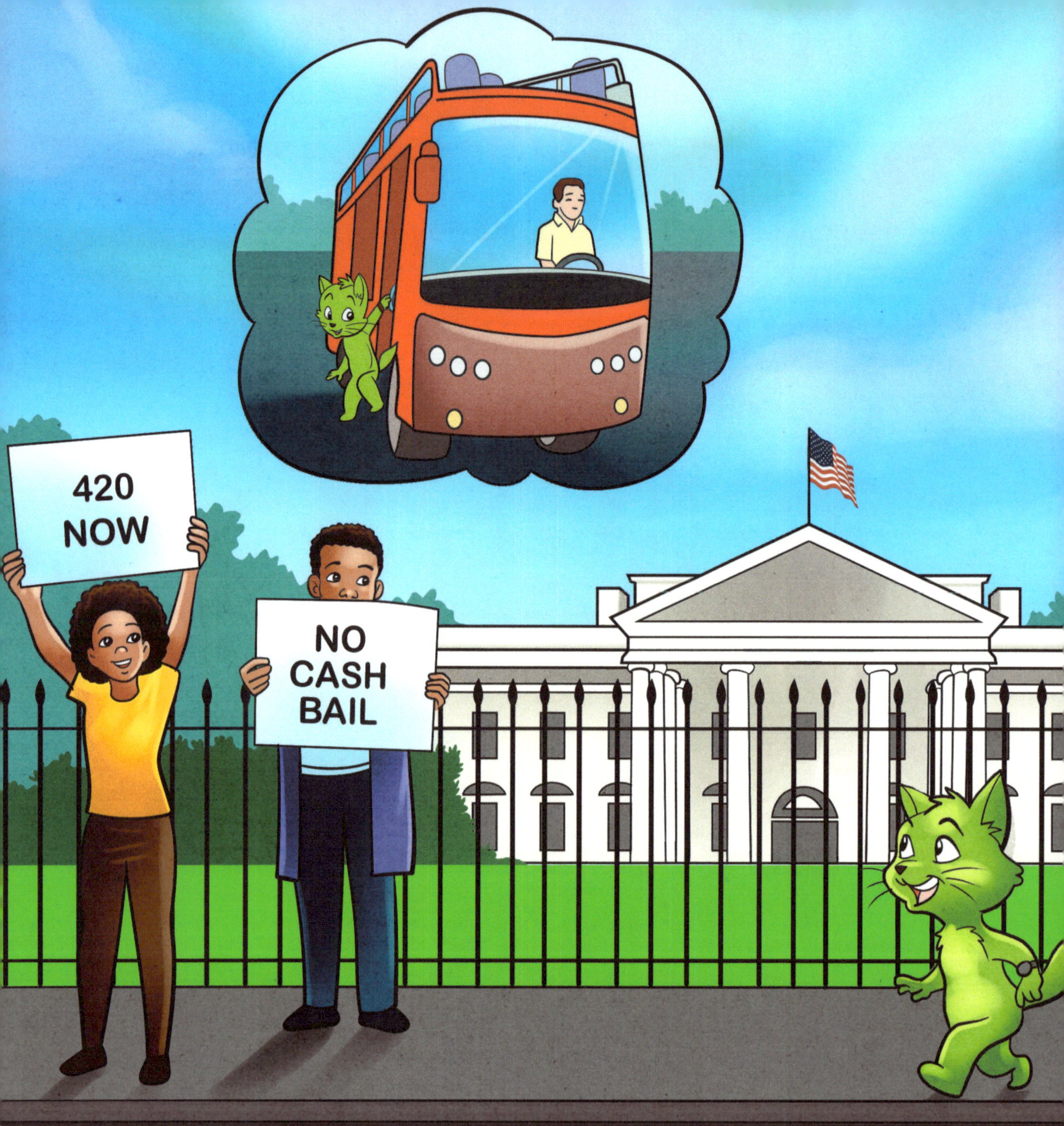

"I think I'll start my tour here at the White House. I see it was built around 1800. Our first president, George Washington, never lived here. But Thomas Jefferson did. Interestingly, both presidents grew hemp in the late 1700's. It has been the home of the President of the United States ever since. Gee, I wonder if President Joe Biden is home?"

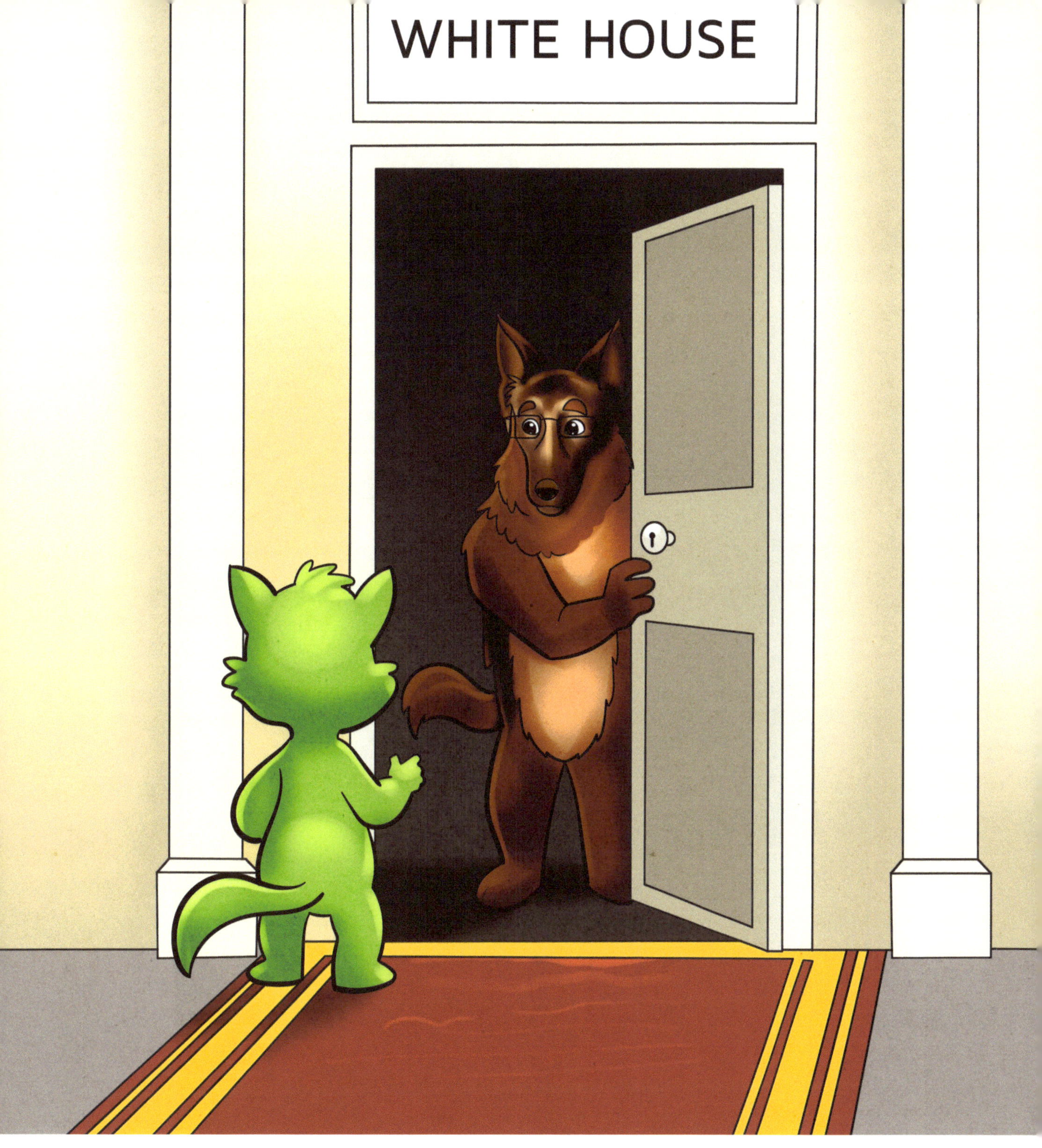

Knock, knock, knock!

"Hi, can I help you?"

"Yes, my name is Cannabis the Cat, and I'm here in Washington, DC this week to talk to very important people about marijuana. Is the President home?" asks Cannabis.

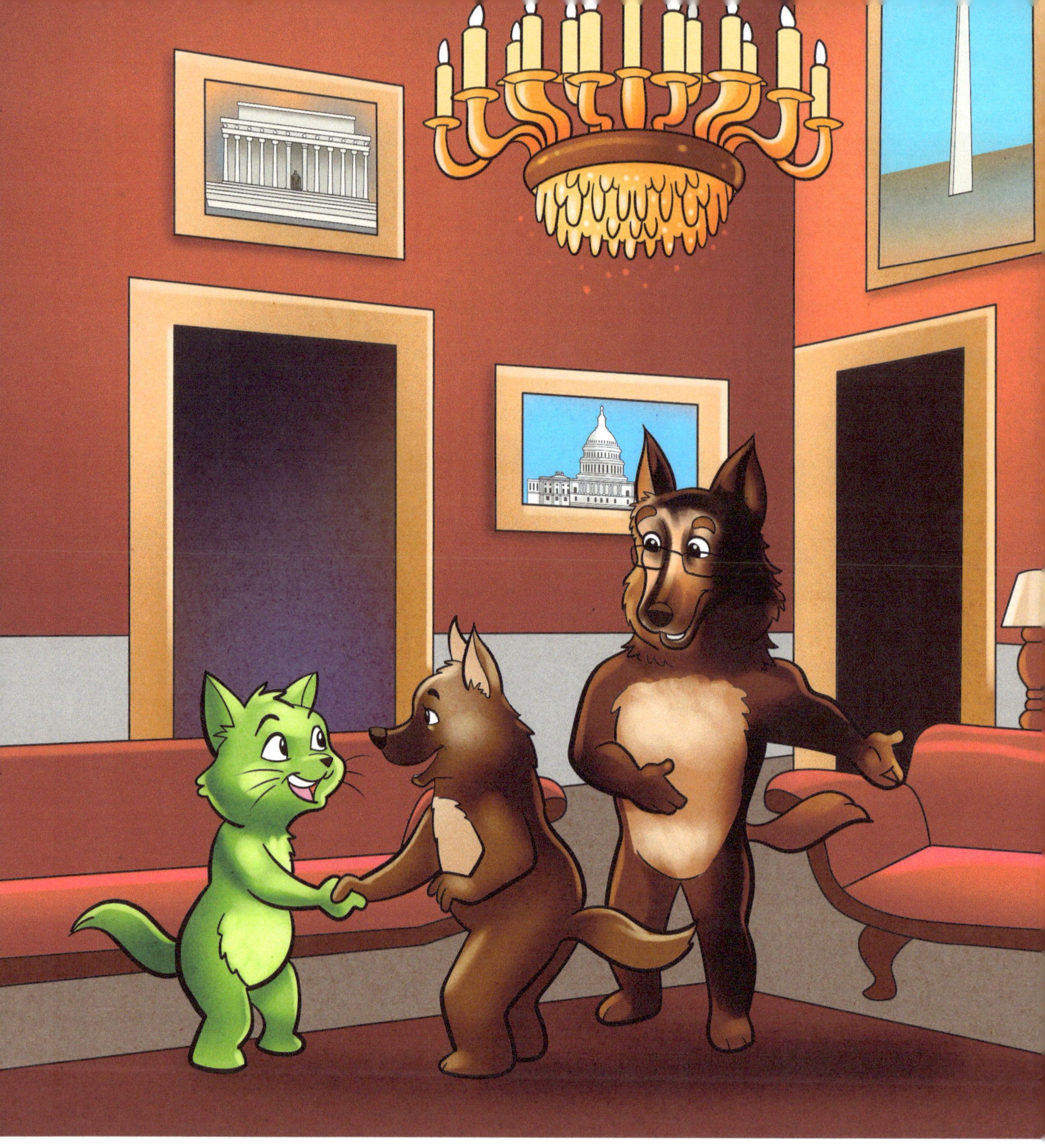

"No, I'm sorry. He is not," replies a German Shepherd dog named Major. "He is away working on very important business. Champ and I keep an eye on the house when Joe is gone. Please come in."

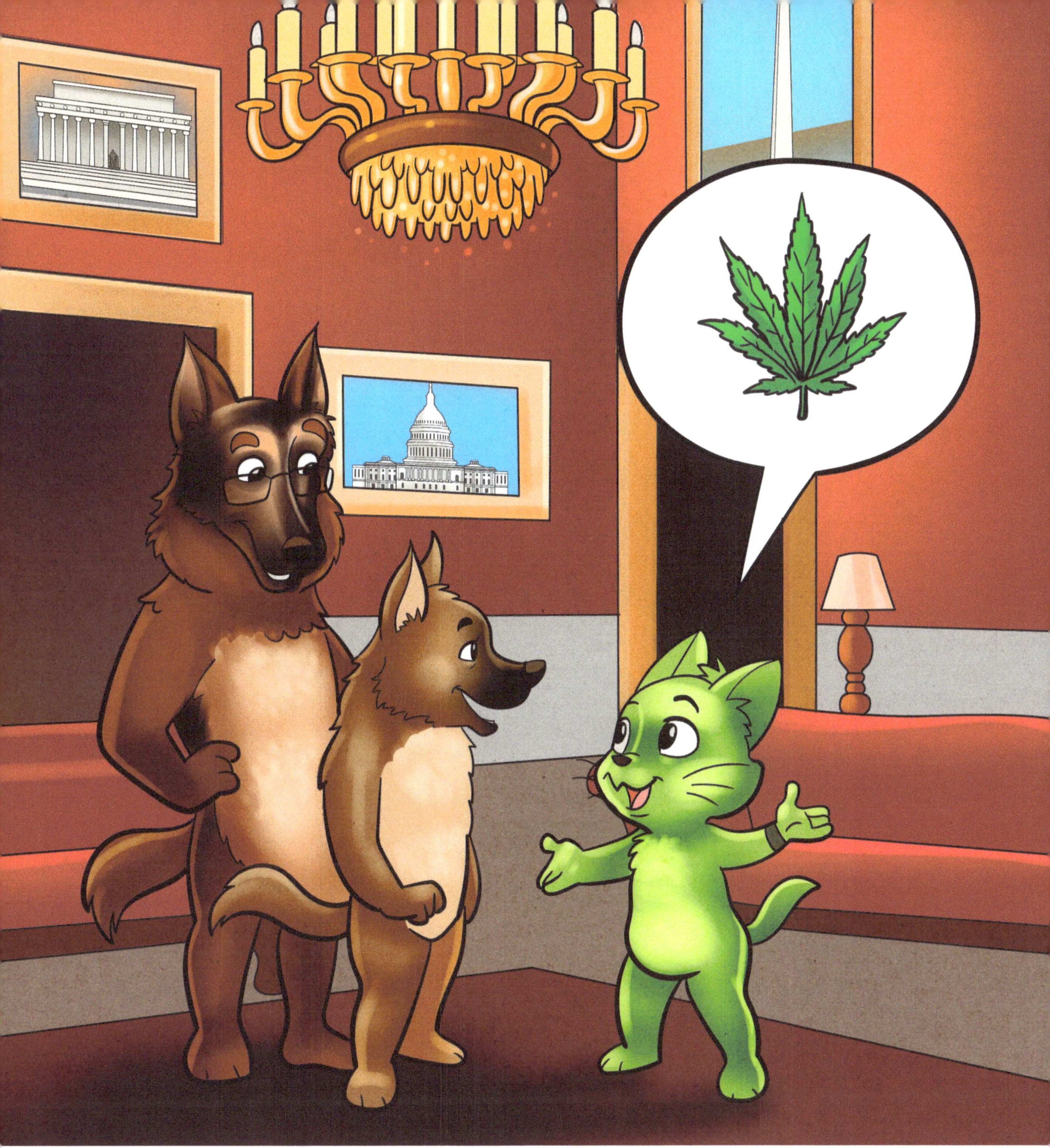

"I'm curious to learn more about marijuana," says Major.
"Me too," says Champ.
"Well, first off it's a plant. It comes from a seed, and it's been around for thousands of years," says cannabis.

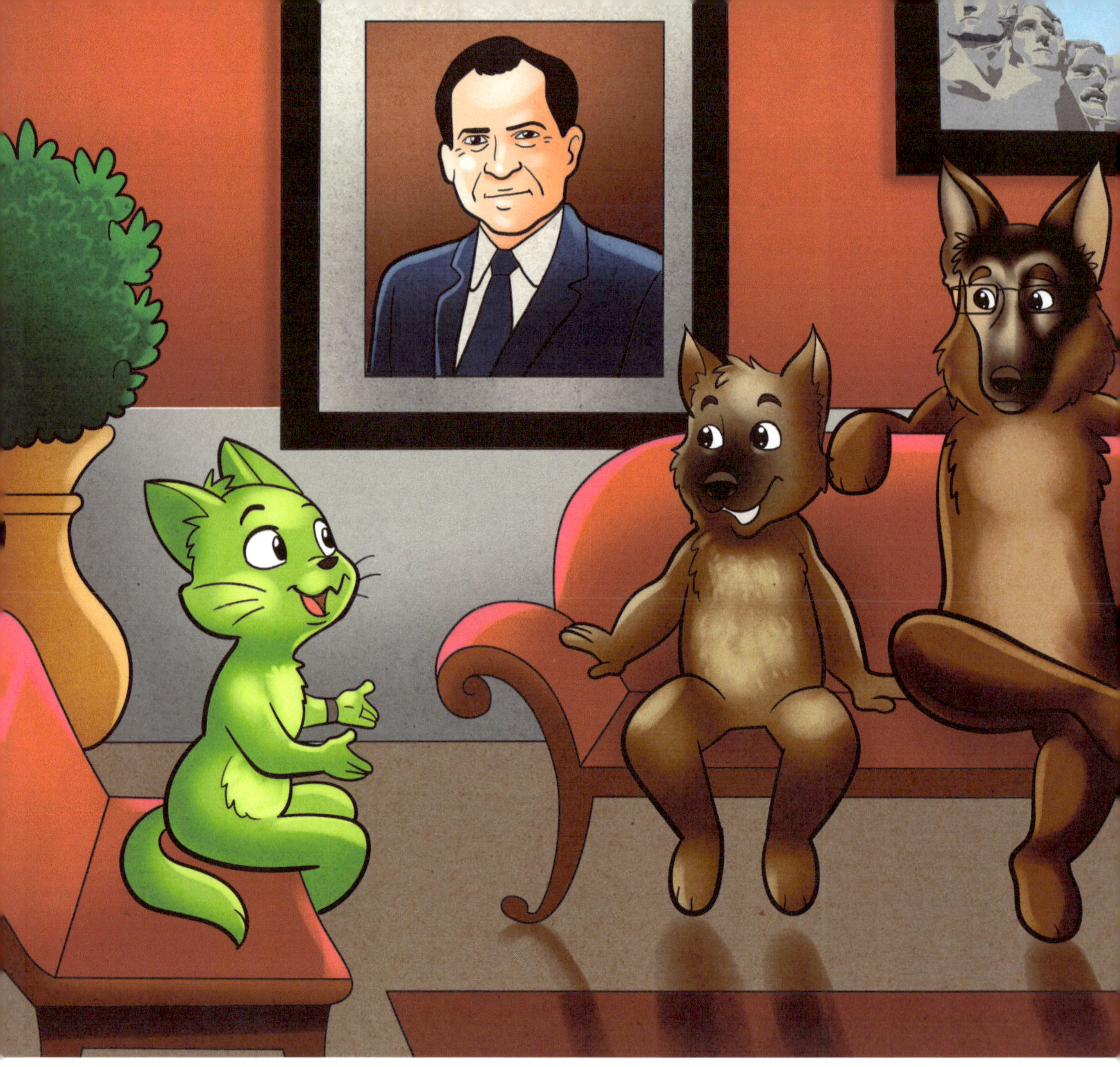

"About a hundred years ago, the United States began outlawing the hemp plant. By 1970, President Richard Nixon declared that marijuana had no medicinal value. He classified marijuana as a schedule one drug. The government then created the idea that marijuana was a gateway drug to more harmful drugs, like heroin and cocaine.

"It was the beginning of the war on drugs. The United States would begin to put millions of Americans in prison for possessing weed and continues to do so today. We still jail 500,000 Americans annually for marijuana possession.

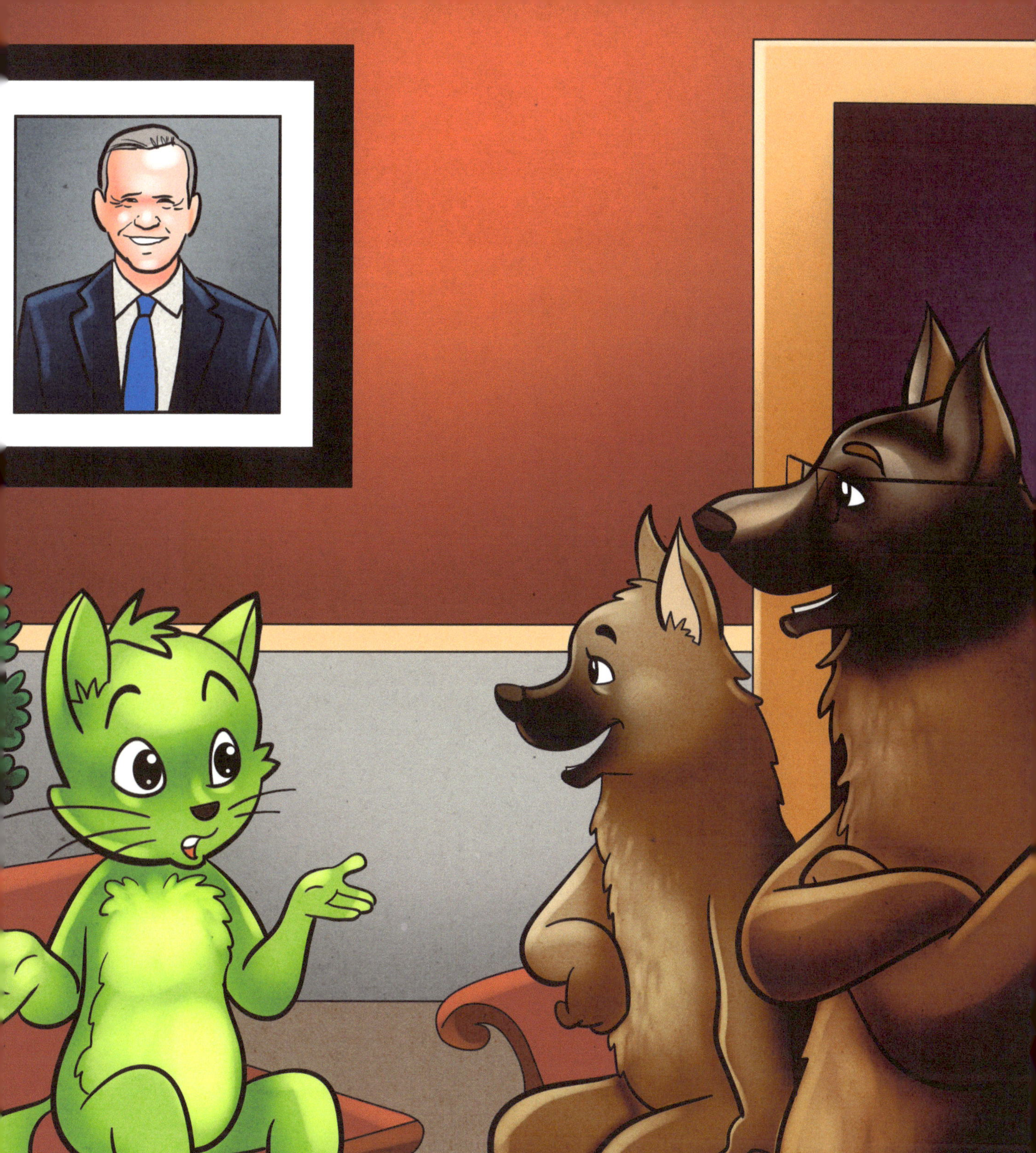

"In reality, people use marijuana in place of dangerous drugs like opiates and cocaine. Marijuana has also been proven to be useful for those who are recovering from alcoholism.

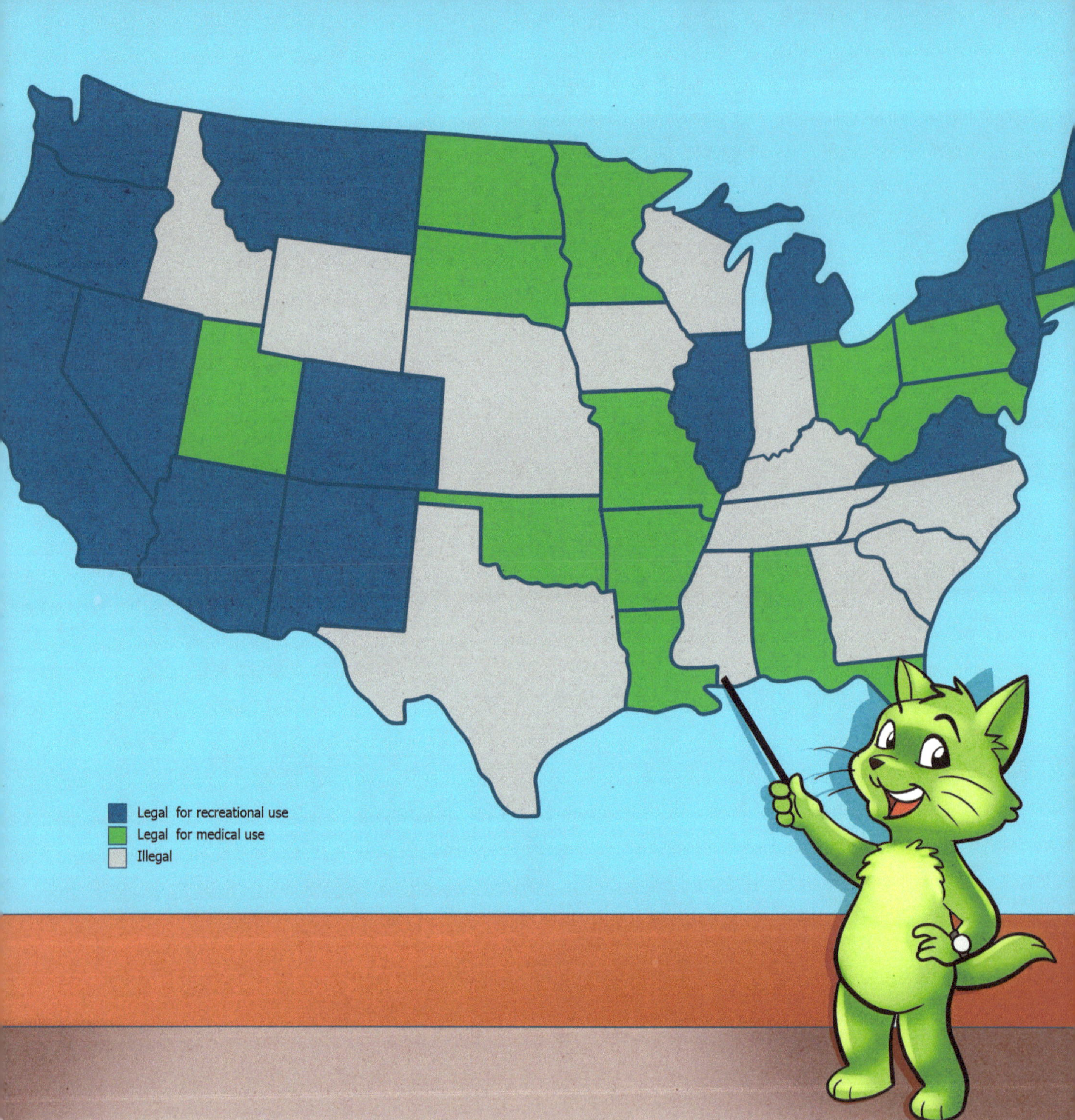

"Today, 37 states allow people to use marijuana for epilepsy, cancer, AIDS, insomnia, PTSD, and pain control. Even for recreational use."

"Wait a minute," says Champ. "We have fifty states. 50 minus 37 equals 13. What about the 13 states where marijuana is still illegal?"

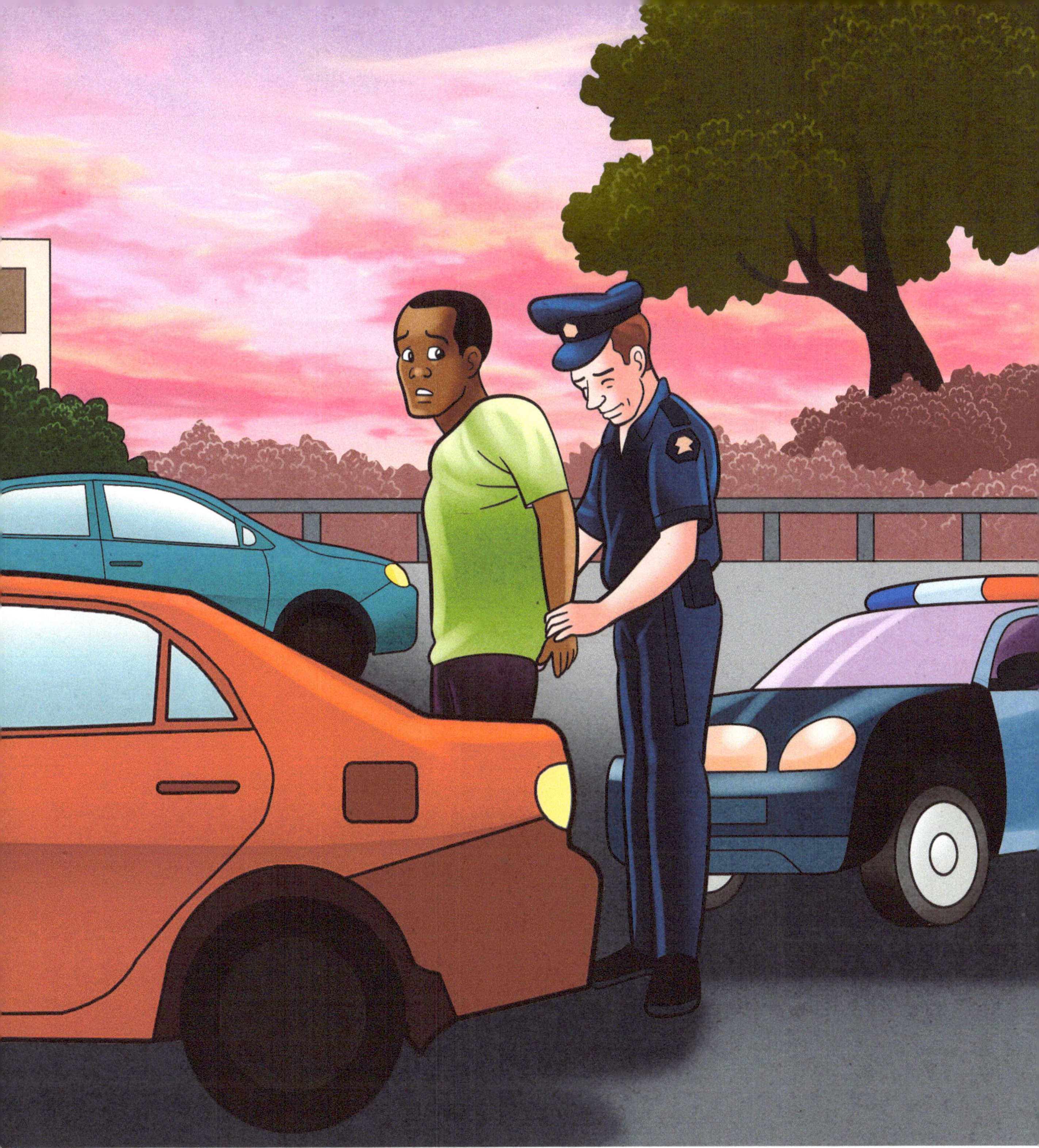

"That's why I'm here in DC," says Cannabis. "We still put people in jail for having weed, especially people of color. They are arrested nearly four times as often as white people for having marijuana."

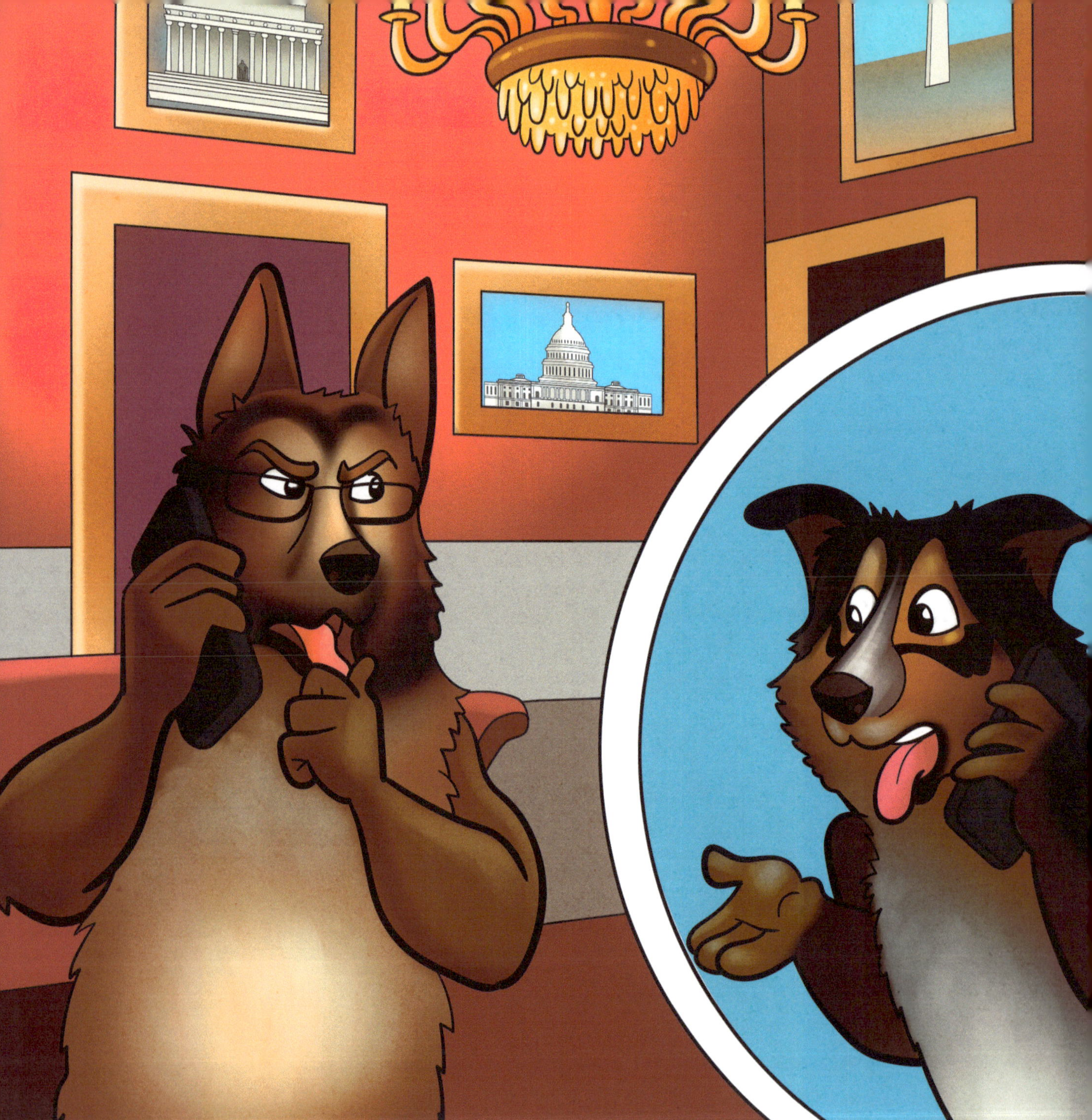

About that time, the telephone rings.

"Hello, you've reached the White House, Major speaking. Hi, Harley, how are you? What? Oh no! Okay, I understand. I'll see what I can do. Bye now." Major hangs up the phone.

"What did Harley want?" asks Champ.

"He said Marlon Bundo is missing! He's afraid Marlon ran away!"

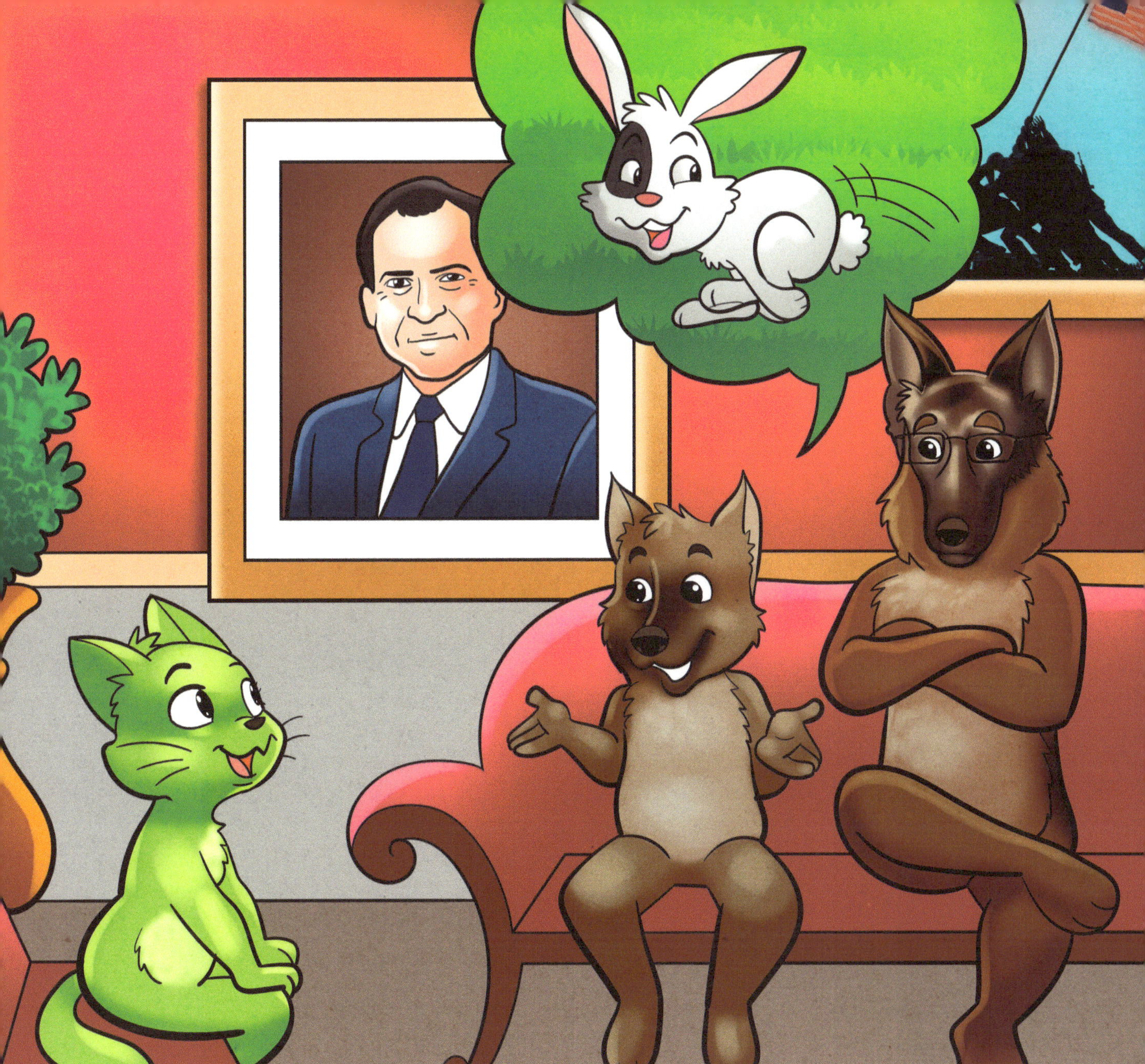

"Who's Marlon Bundo?" asks Cannabis.

"He's our friend the bunny rabbit who lives with Vice President Mike Pence and his family," says Champ. "Ever since the loss in the election, Marlon has never been the same. He knows if he moves back to Indiana where the Pence family is from, he'll never have another birthday cake again. All Marlon would ever talk about was no more cake for his birthday parties, ever again."

"I'm confused. I don't understand," says Cannabis.

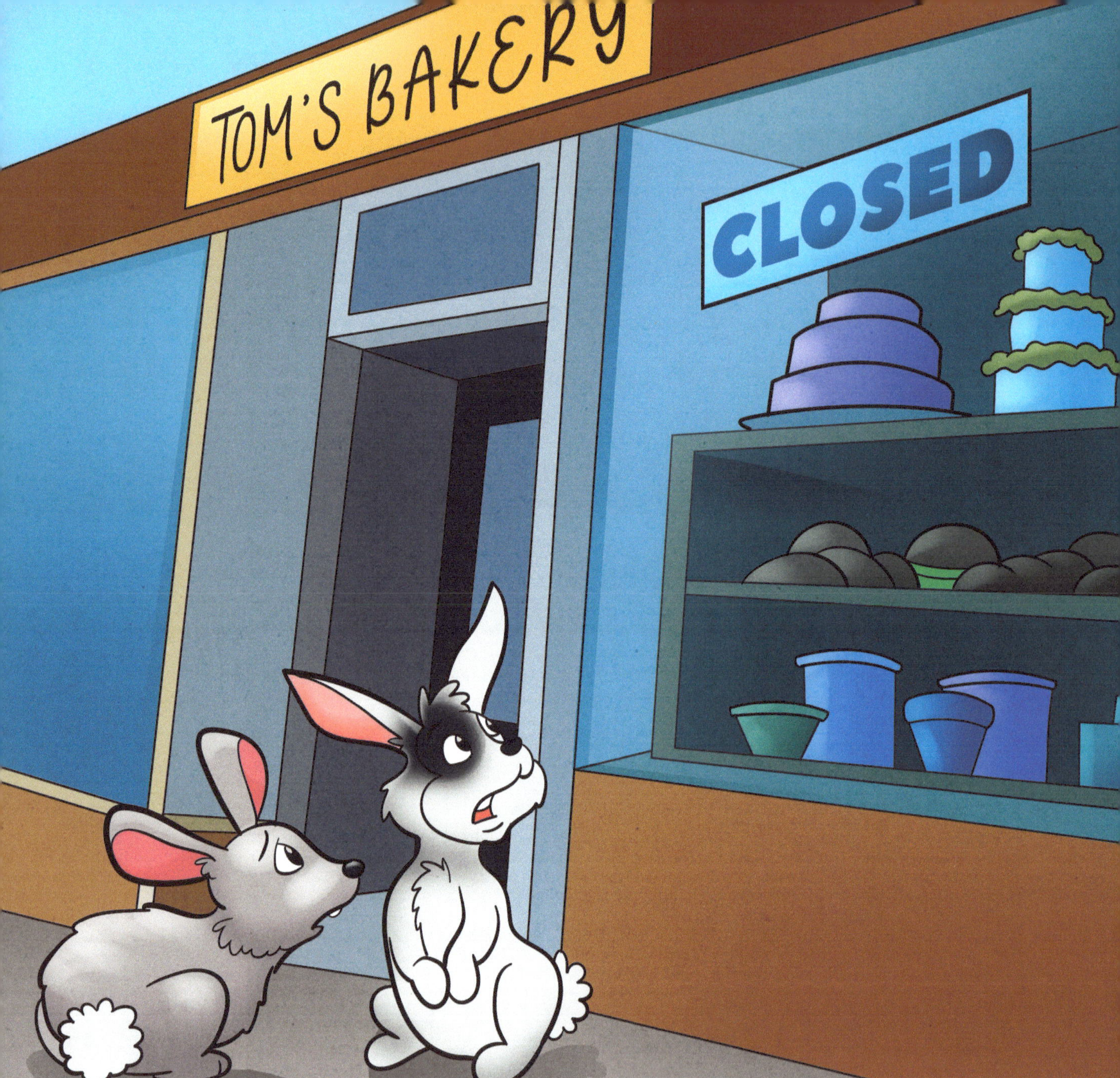

"Well, ever since Marlon married his bunny rabbit friend, Arthur, Vice President Pence and Marlon have not talked," says Champ.

"I still don't understand," says Cannabis.

"Marlon and Arthur are boy bunny rabbits, and some humans are funny about that sort of thing," says Major.

"And if they won't bake a wedding cake for a gay couple in Indiana, they certainly won't bake a birthday cake for two gay bunny rabbits either," adds Champ.

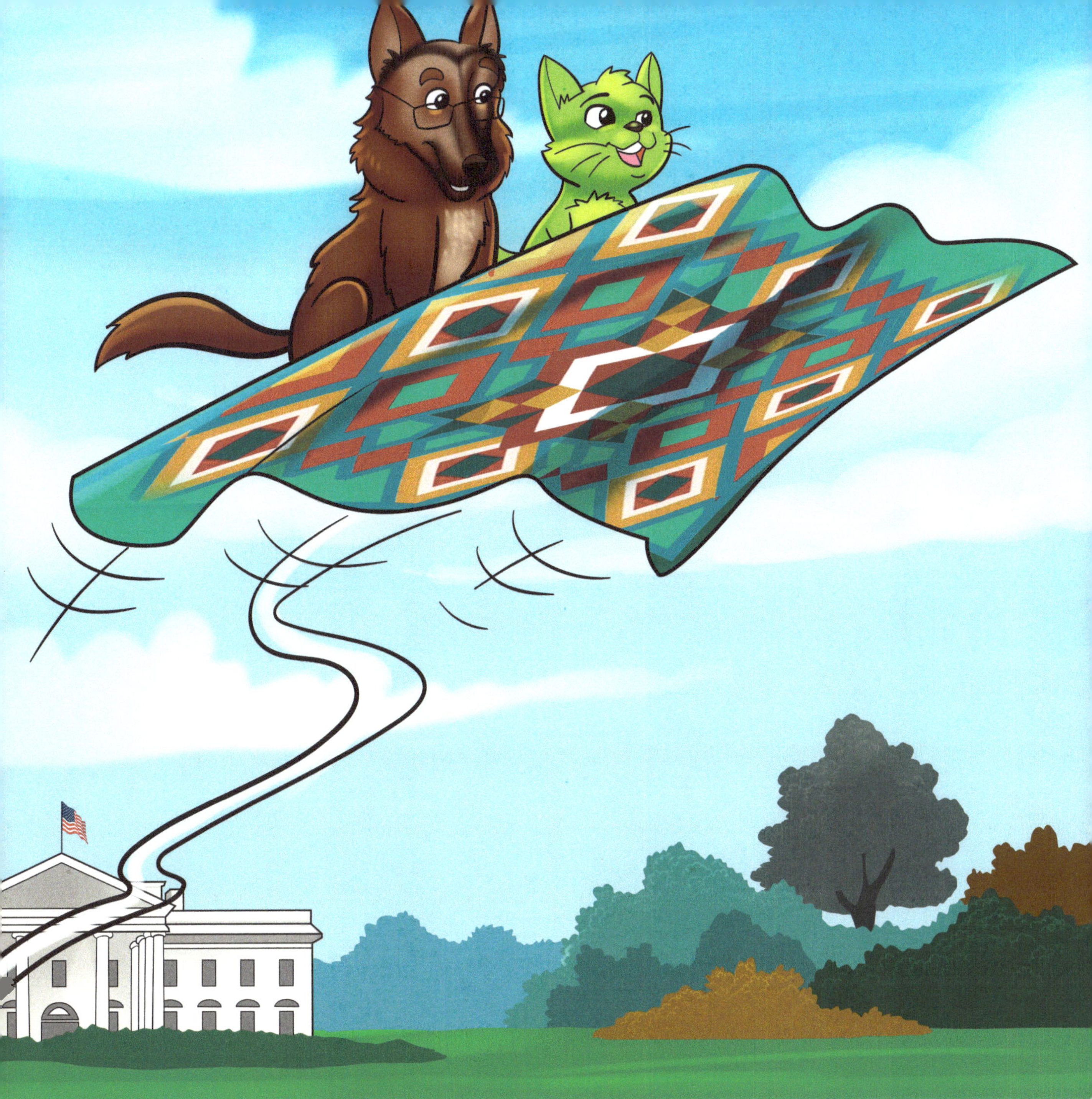

"Now I understand. I wanna help. Let's jump on my magic hemp carpet and fly around DC, and maybe we can find Marlon Bundo!" says Cannabis.

"That sounds like a great plan!" says Major. So Major and Cannabis jump on the magic hemp carpet and fly off in search of Marlon Bundo.

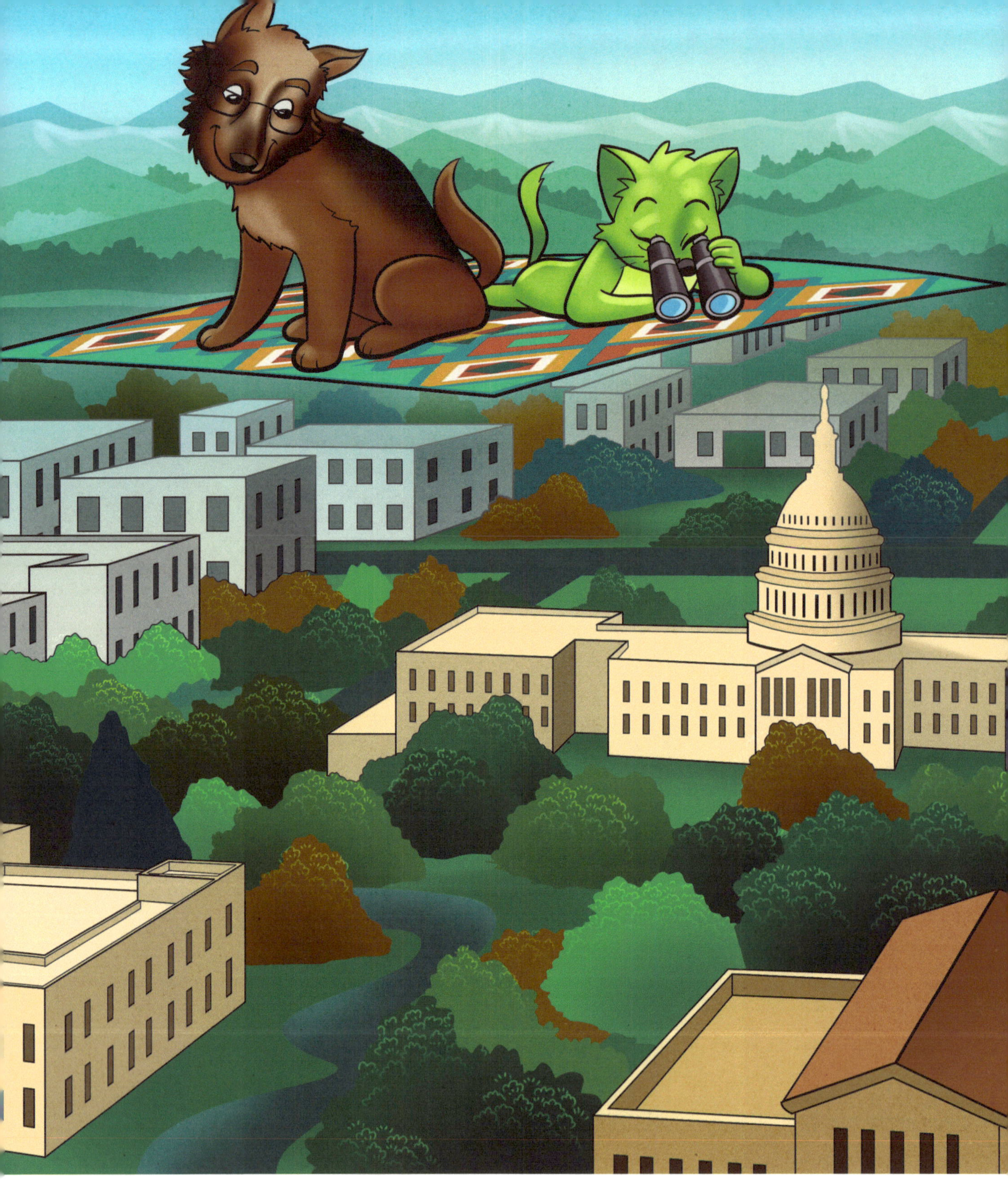

Major and Cannabis fly throughout the sky, looking everywhere for Marlon Bundo.

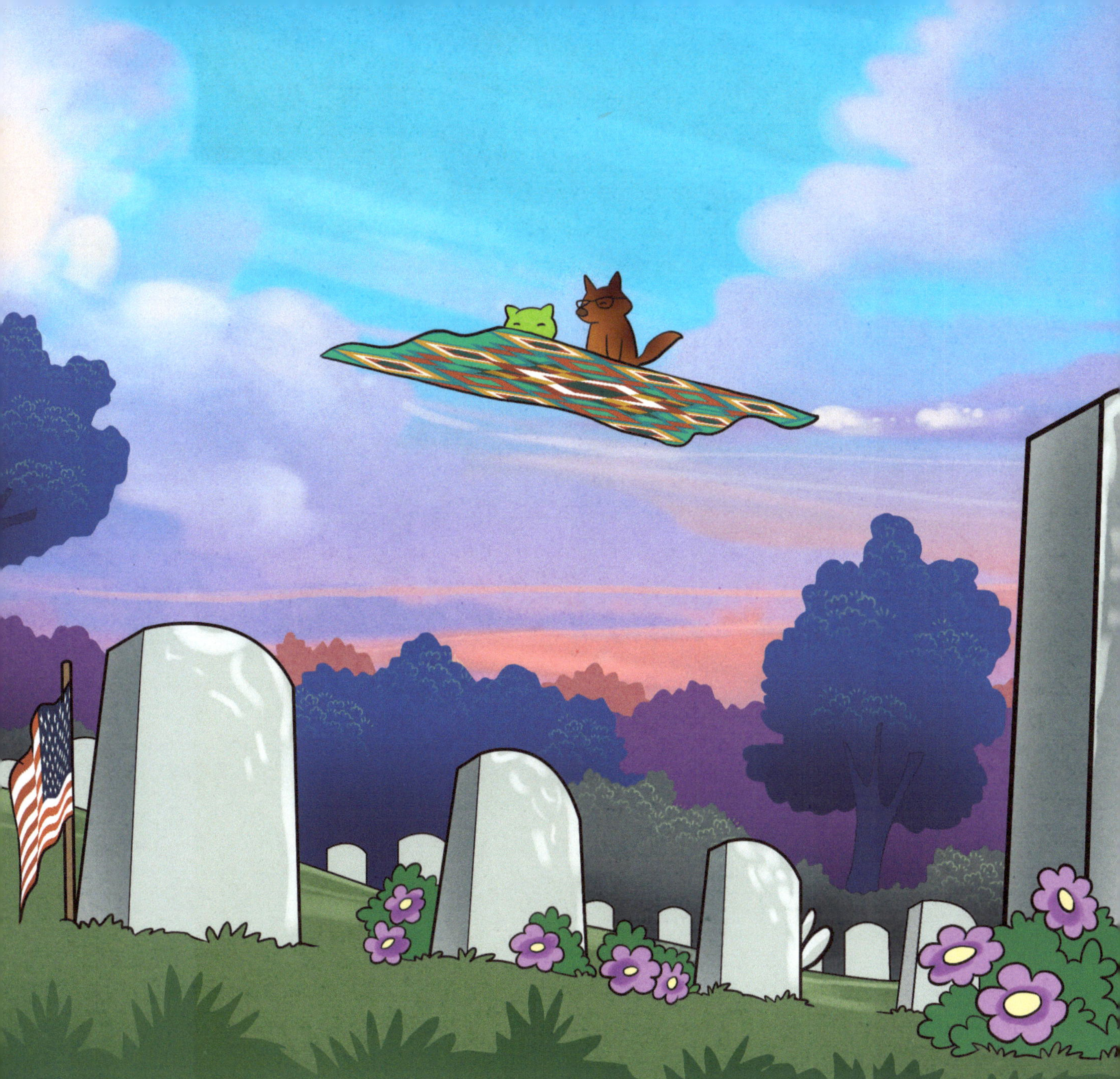

"Wow! What's that over there?" asks Cannabis.

"That is Arlington Cemetery," says Major. "American service men and women whose lives ended while serving our country are buried there. John F. Kennedy and William Howard Taft are the only two presidents buried in Arlington Cemetery.

"Cannabis, take us down. I think I see a set of rabbit ears!" Seconds later Cannabis and Major land at Arlington Cemetery.

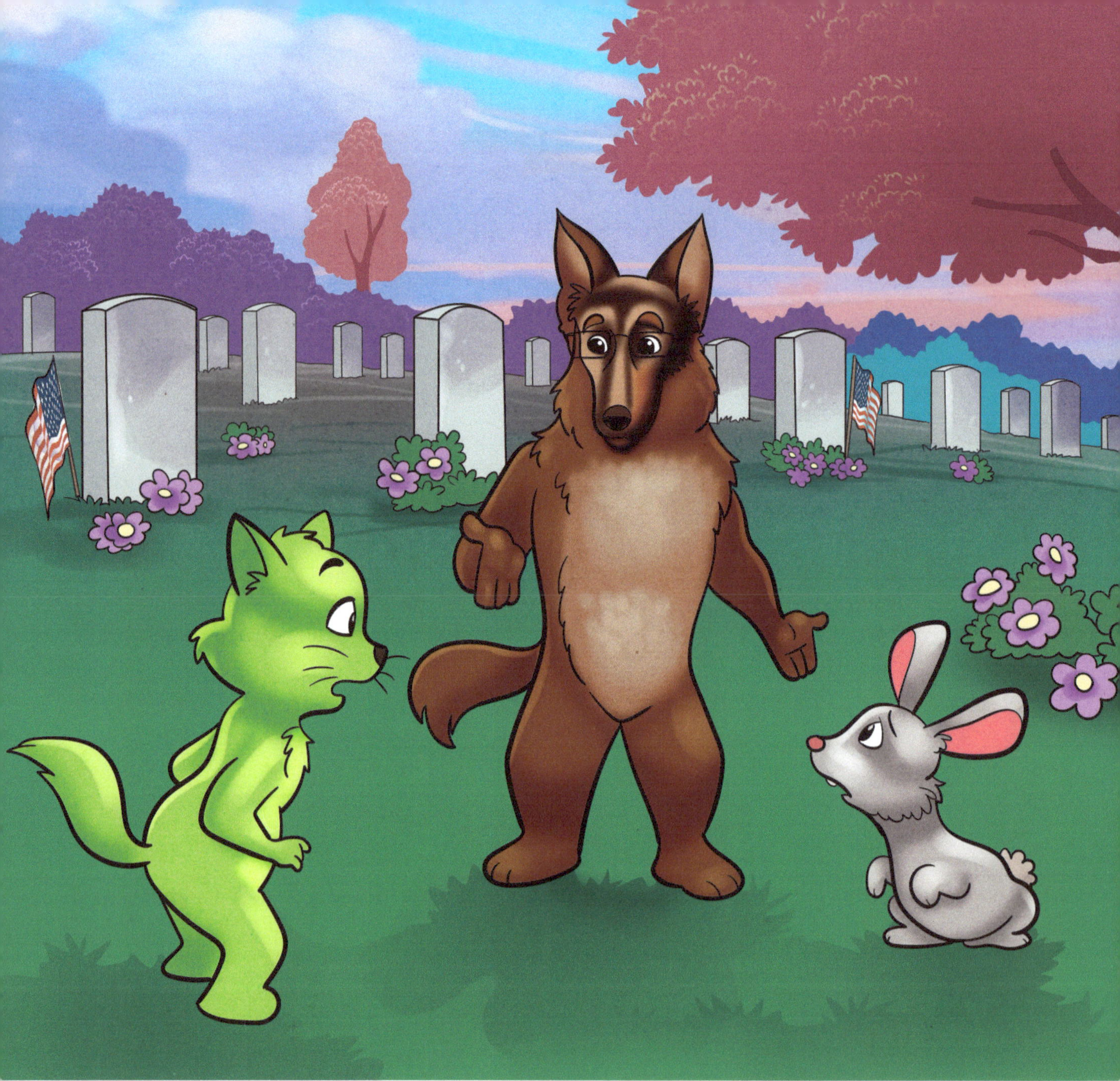

"Oh! It's my rabbit friend, Arthur. Have you seen Marlon Bundo?" asks Major.

"No, I haven't," replies Arthur. "I just know that Marlon has been very sad. He does not want to move back to Indiana. He has been having bad cake dreams at night. Have you tried the Vice President's house?" asks Arthur.

"No, we haven't, but that sounds like a great idea," says Major.

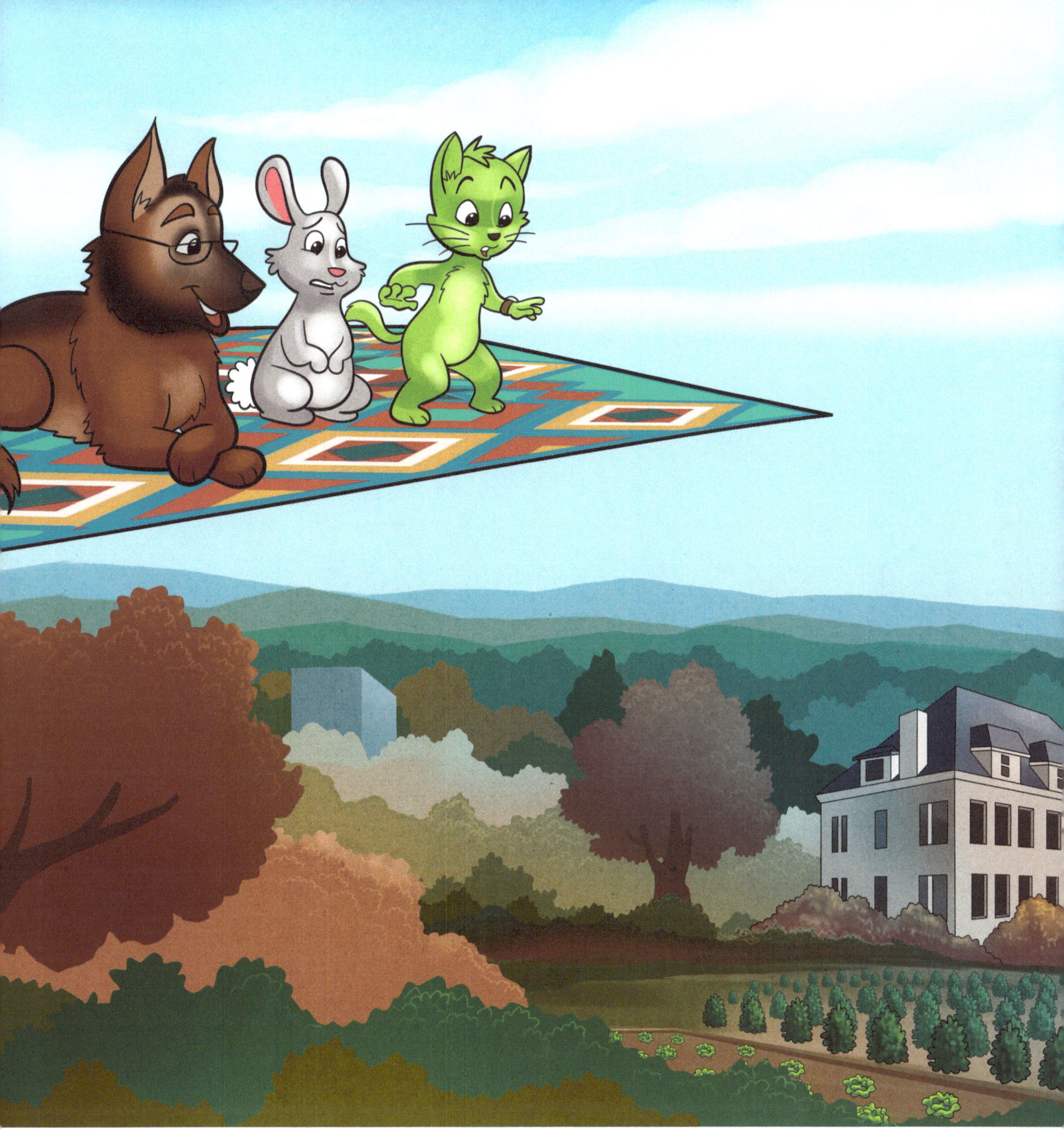

So Major, Arthur, and Cannabis hop on the magic carpet and fly straight to the Naval Observatory, where the Vice President of the United States lives.

"Whee! This is fun, Cannabis! You're the only cat I know who has a magic flying carpet!" yells Arthur.

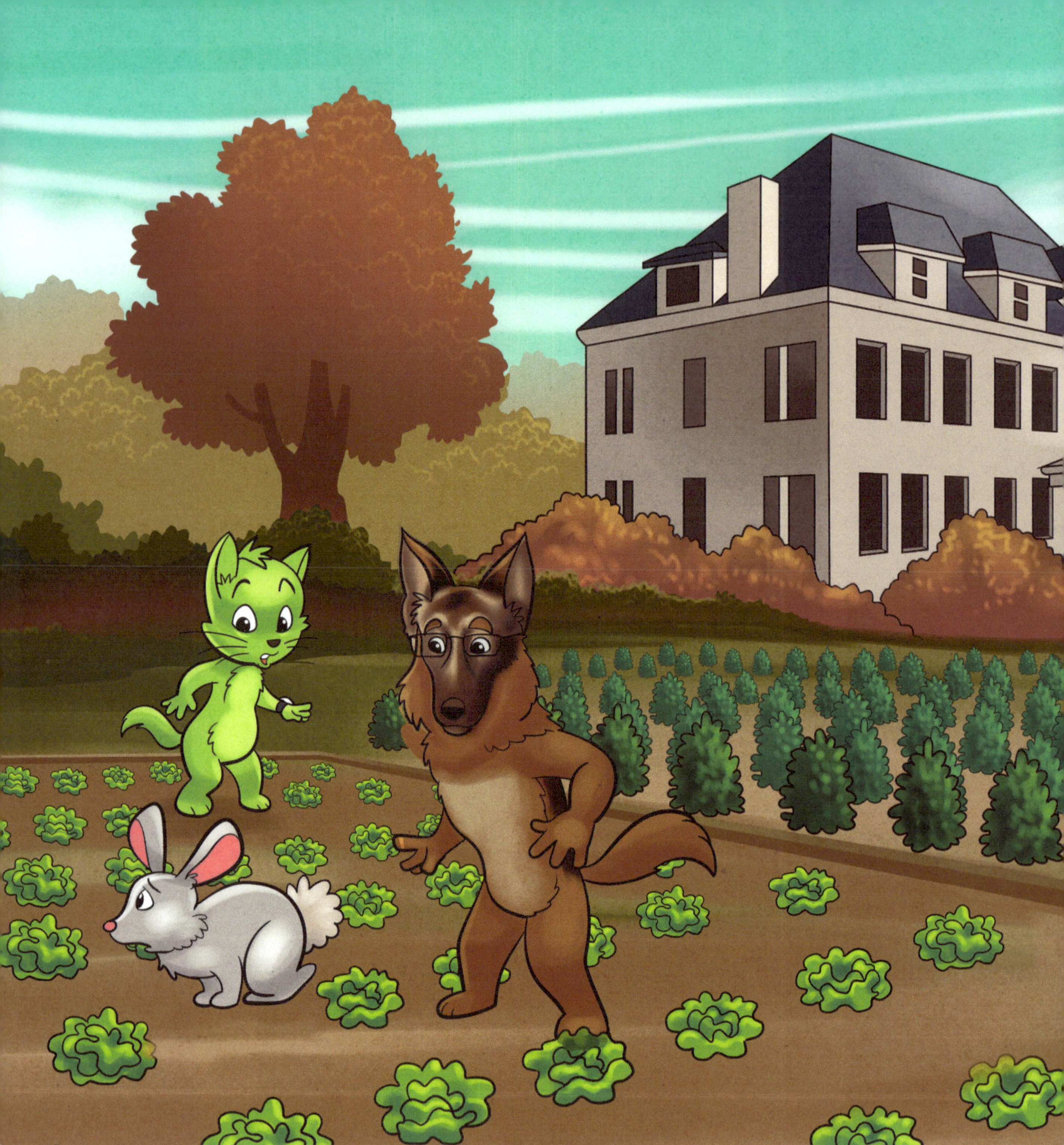

Seconds later, Cannabis, Arthur, and Major arrive at the home of The Vice President of the United States.

"I'm gonna check the vegetable garden," says Arthur. "That's one of Marlon's favorite spots."

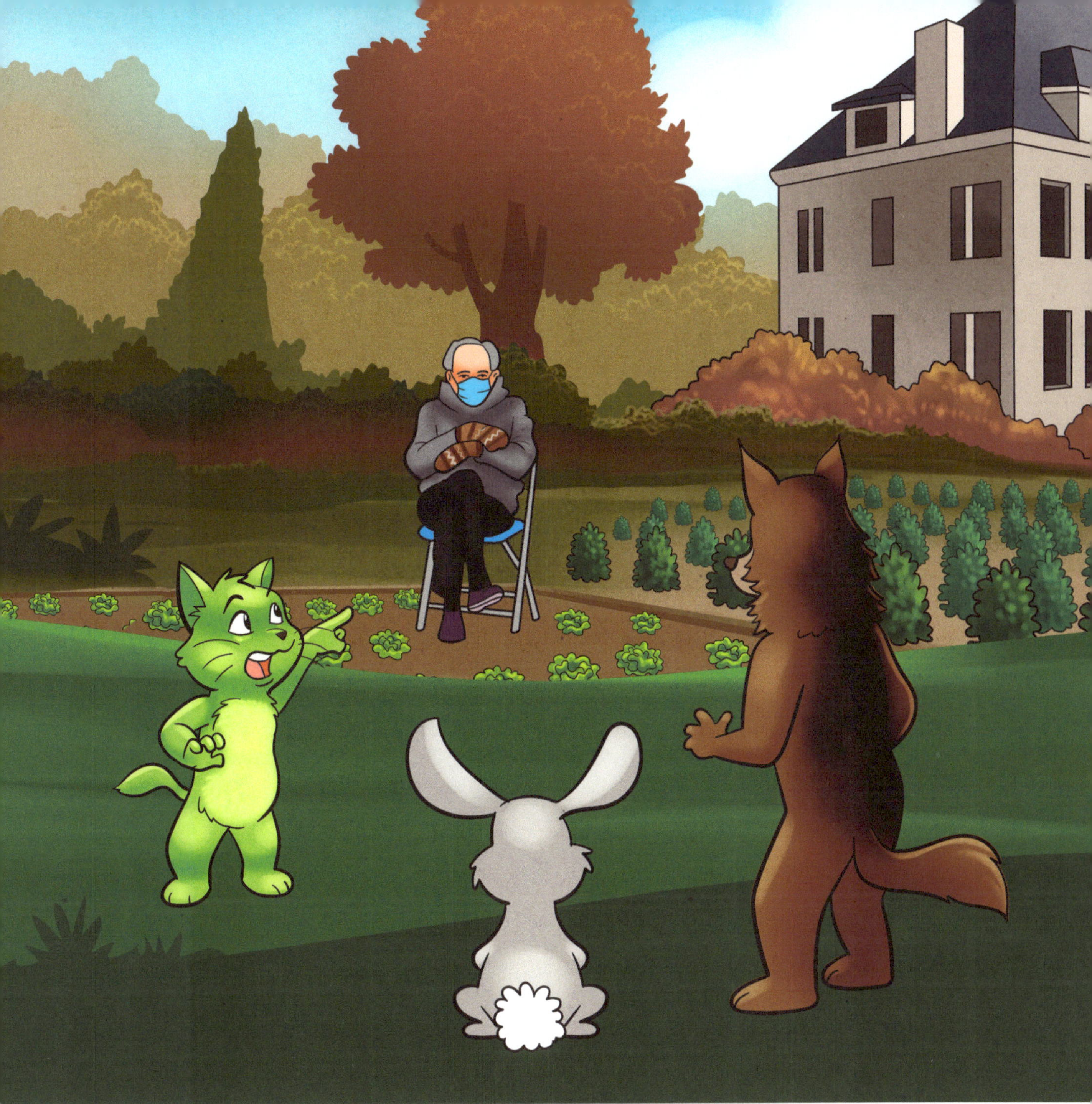

Cannabis and Major walk around the entire house. They look everywhere, and still they see no signs of Marlon Bundo.

Suddenly Cannabis sees a man sitting on a bench. "Who is that?" asks Cannabis.

"Oh, don't worry, Cannabis. That's just Senator Bernie Sanders from Vermont. He, too, is impatient about marijuana legalization!"

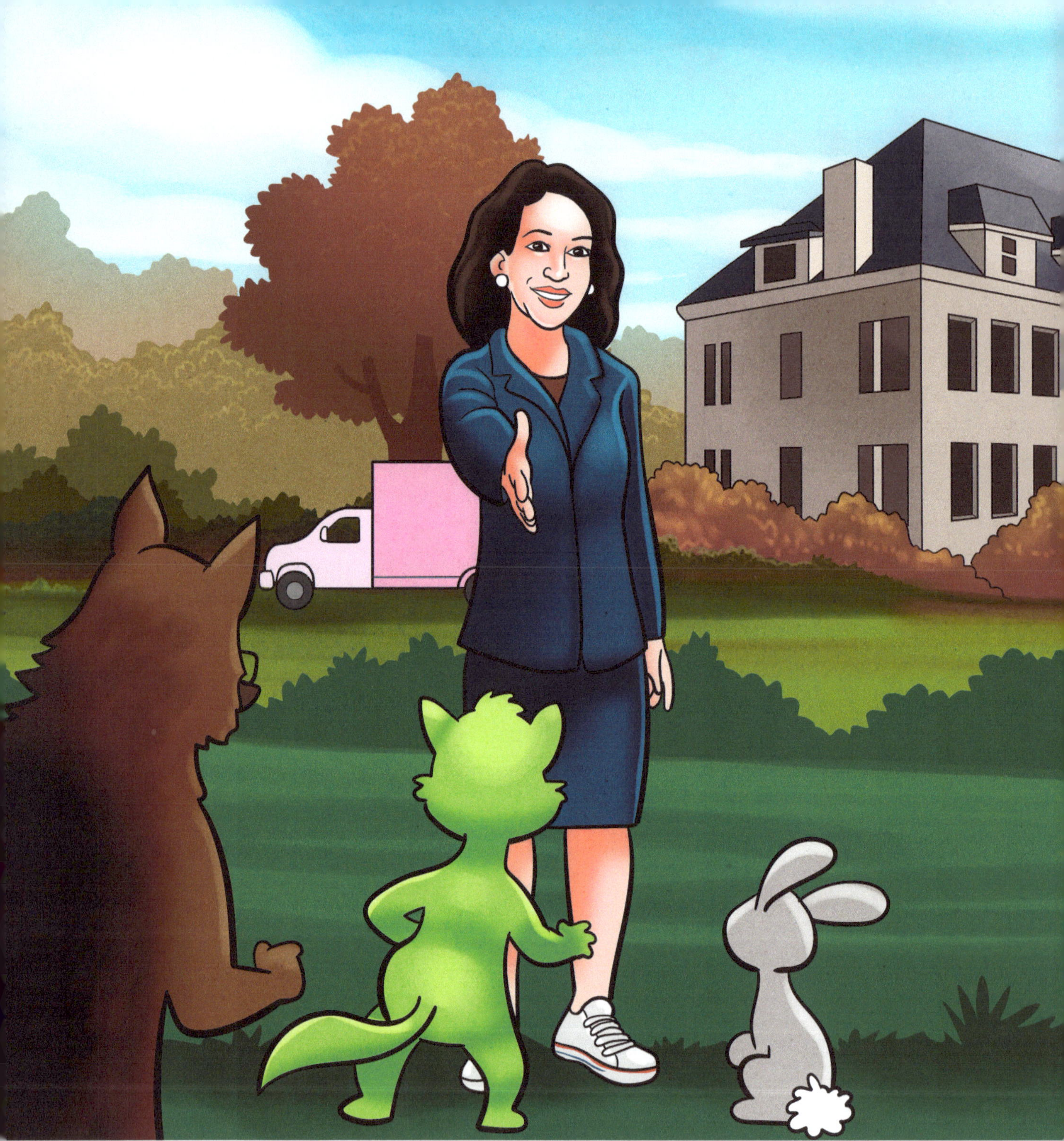

Just then Cannabis looks up, and he is greeted by a startling surprise. "Hello, I'm Kamala Harris, and I am the new Vice President of the United States."

"It's very nice to meet you, Madam Vice President," says Cannabis.

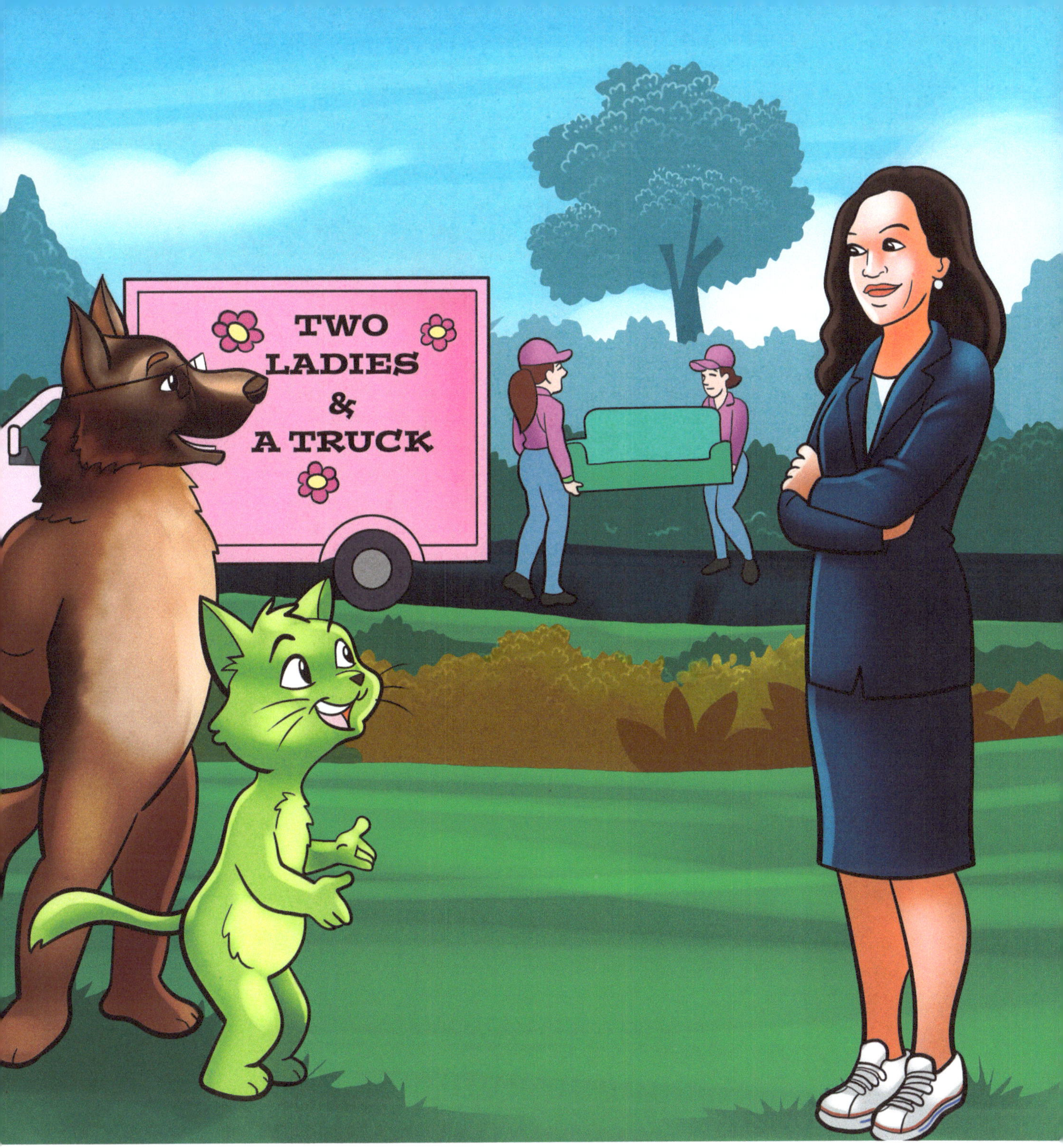

Cannabis quickly jumps into action and thanks the Vice-President for her willingness to legalize marijuana.

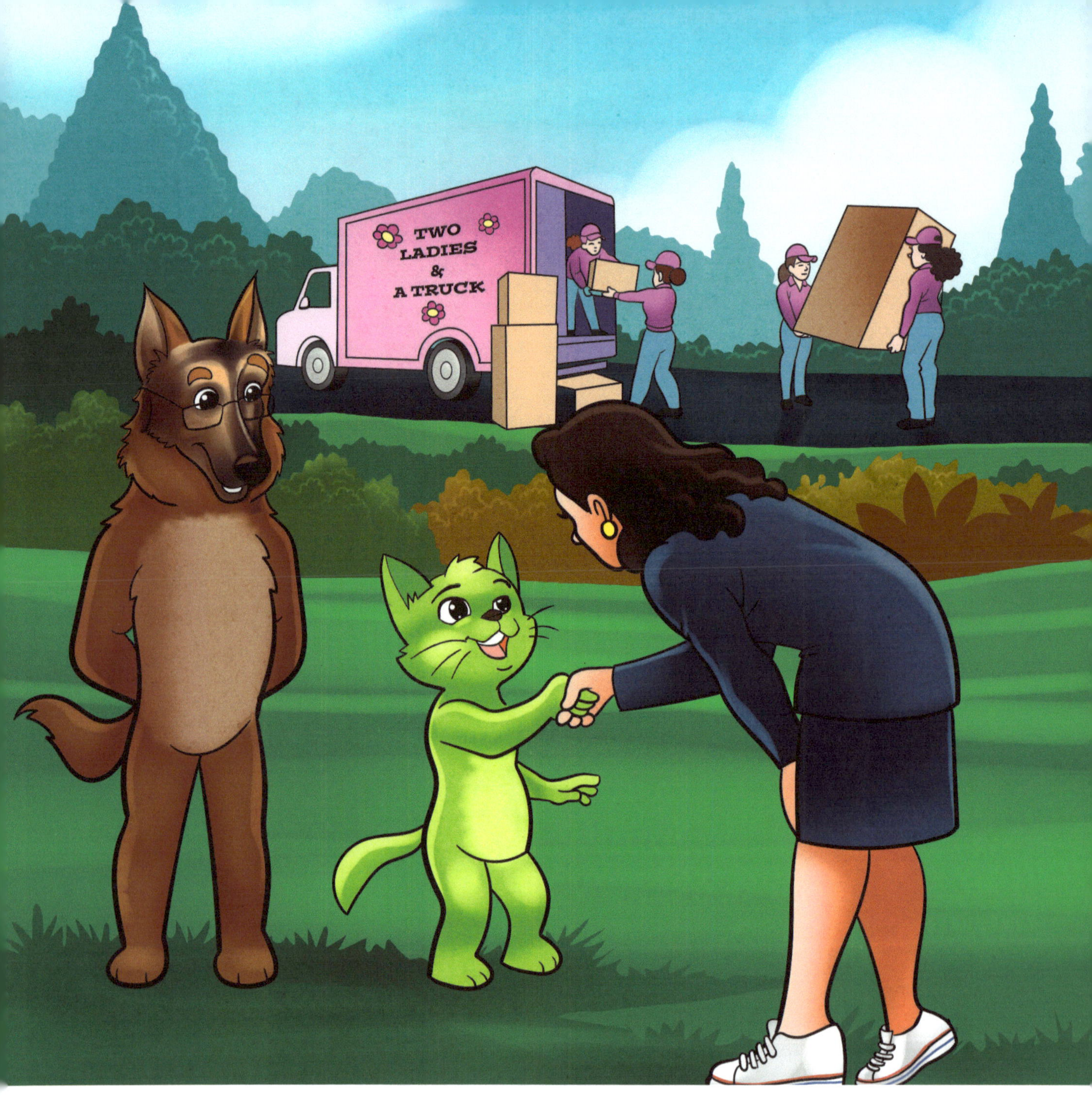

"Don't you worry, Cannabis. We are going to legalize marijuana," says Kamala. "But first, I must get moved into this beautiful old house, and then I will work on very important issues, including marijuana. And remember, Cannabis, we always need more advocates!"

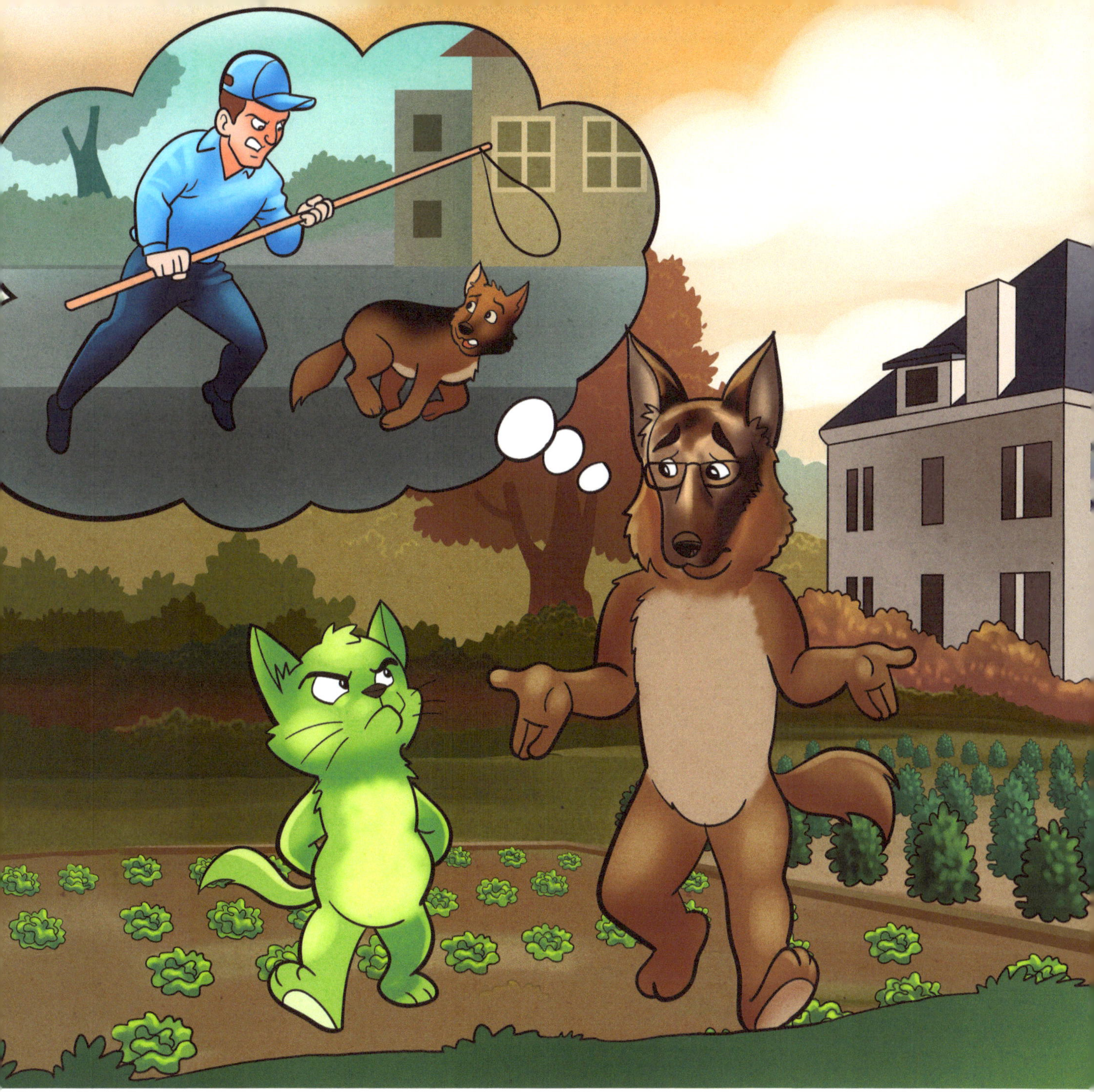

As Cannabis and Major walk back to the vegetable garden, Major comes up with a new idea.

"I think I've got it!" says Major. "There was a time in my life when things were not very good for me. I was down on my luck, and I became homeless. I'll never forget the night the animal catcher found me and took me to the Humane Society.

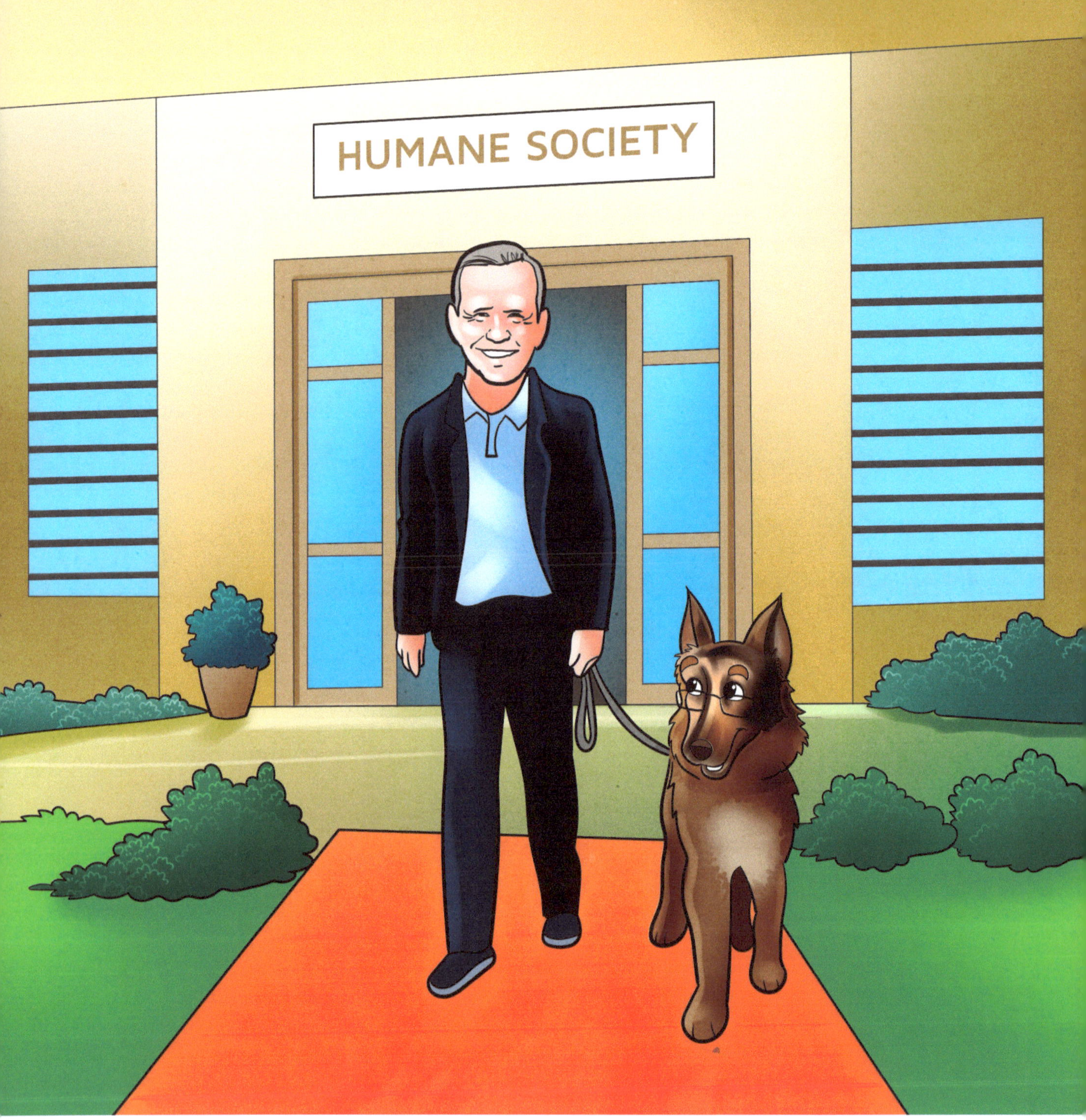

"I was scared at first, but the Humane Society saved my life. They helped me get back on my feet. I'll always be grateful for what they did. In fact, that's where I met Joe. He came to the Humane Society one day and adopted me. It was the best day of my life," says Major.

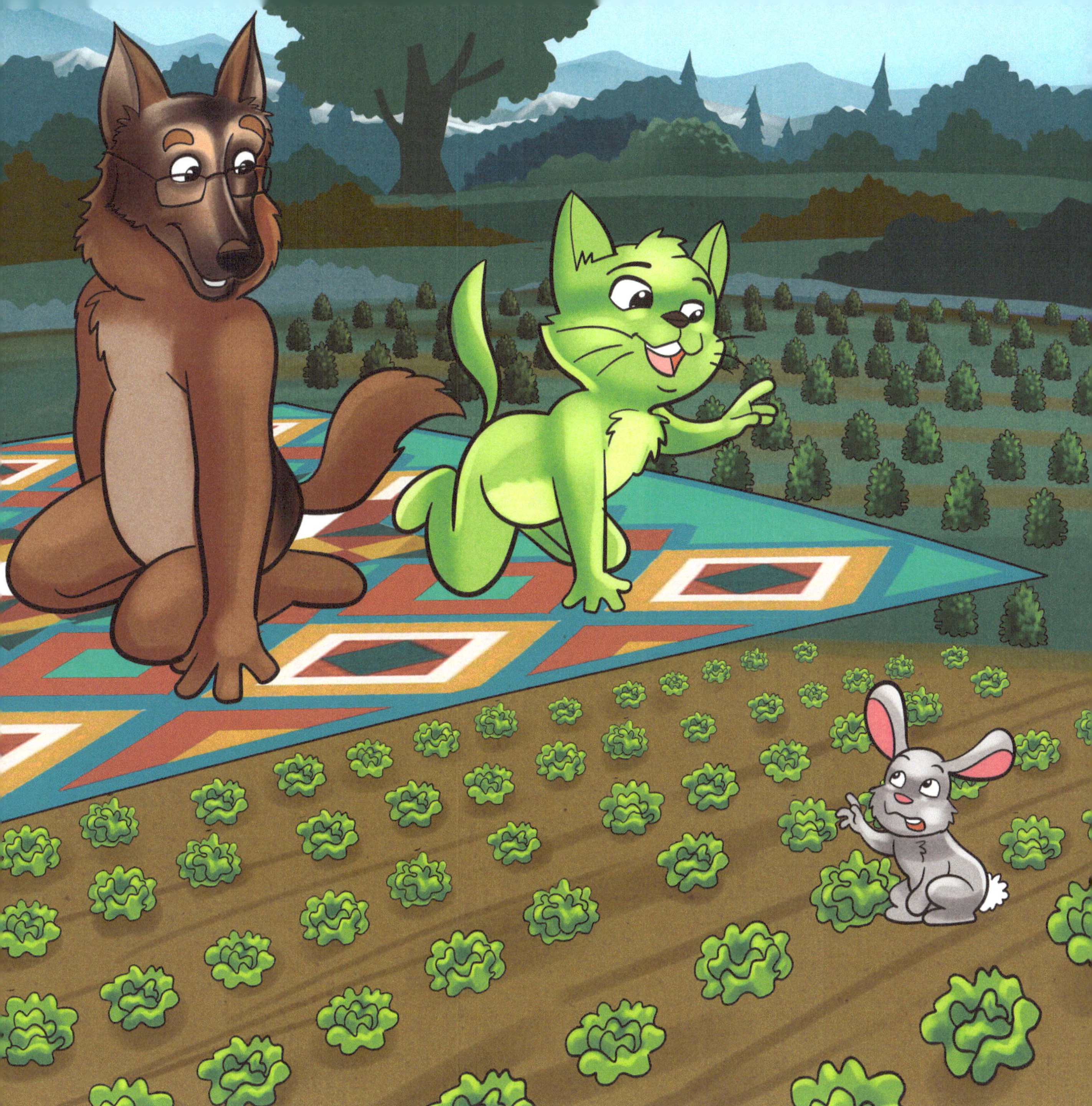

"Perfect! Then it's settled. Let's go check the Humane Society for Marlon!" says Cannabis.

"Okay!" says Major.

"I'll stay here in the vegetable garden just in case Marlon appears," says Arthur.

So Cannabis and Major jump on the magic carpet and fly off for the Humane Society.

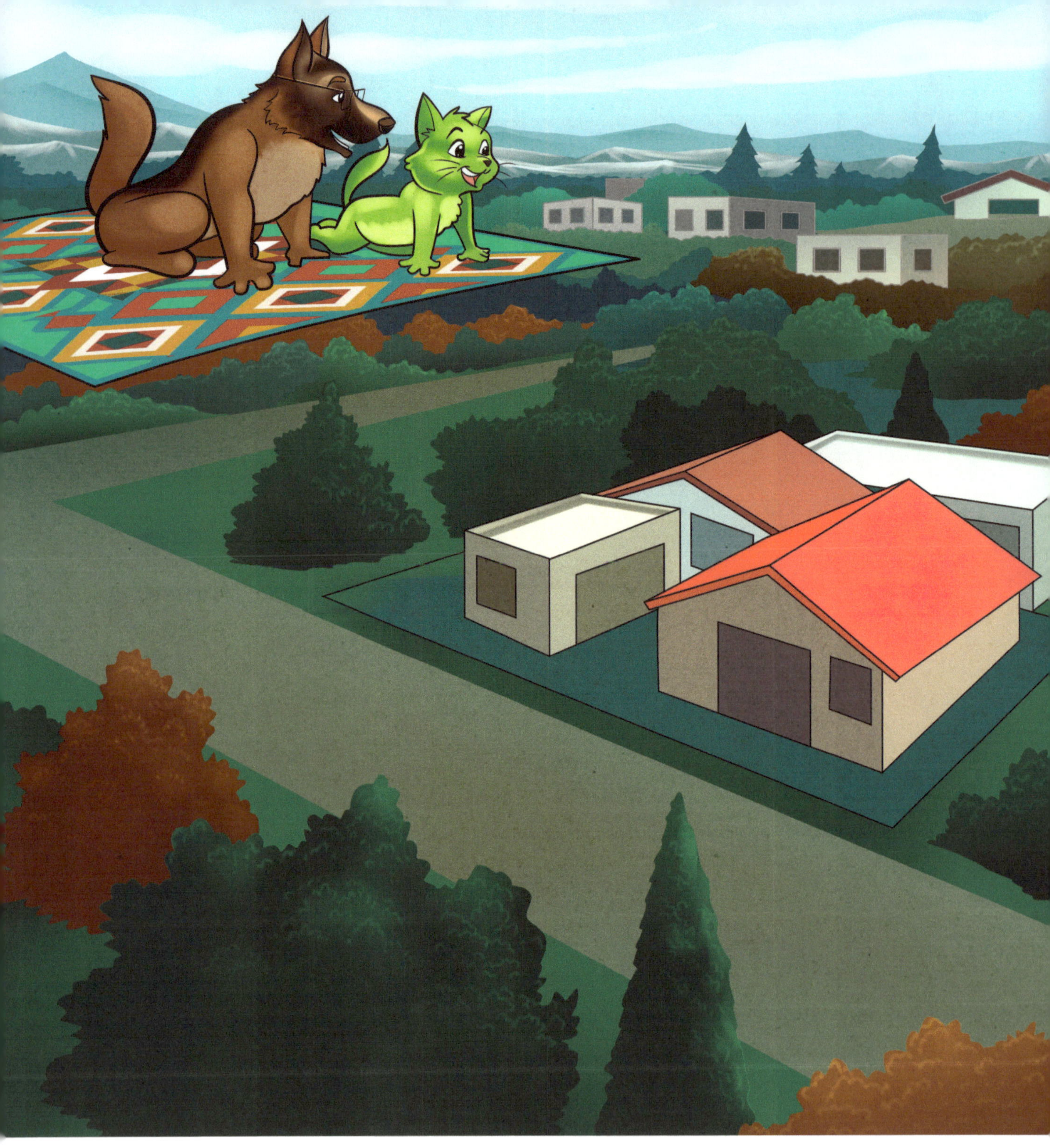

"Washington, DC sure is beautiful from up high!" says Major.
"Yes, it sure is. Look over there! It's the Washington, DC Humane Society," says Cannabis.

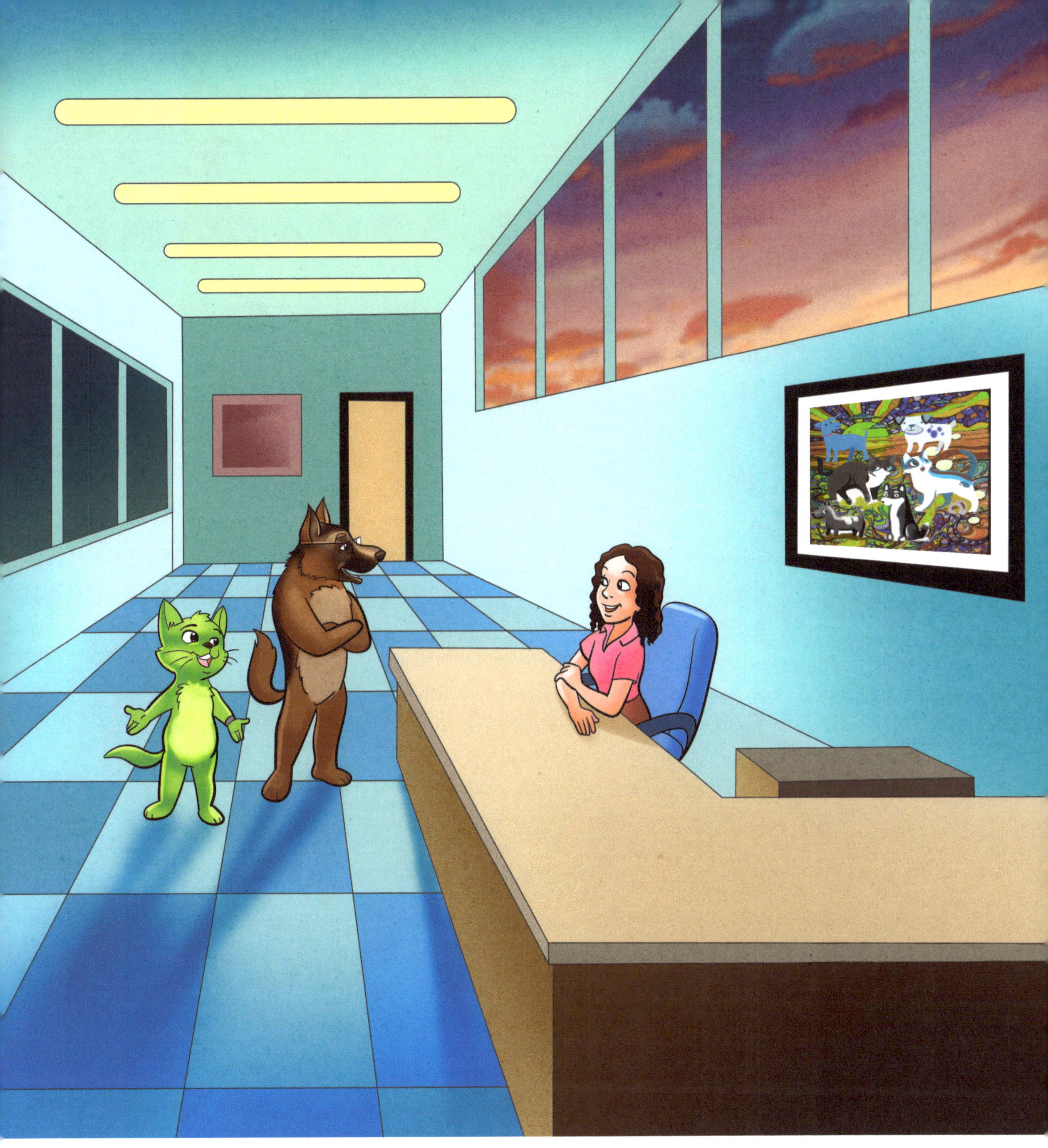

"Hello, we're looking for our friend, Marlon Bundo. He is a friendly bunny rabbit with black and white spots. Have you seen him?" asks Cannabis.

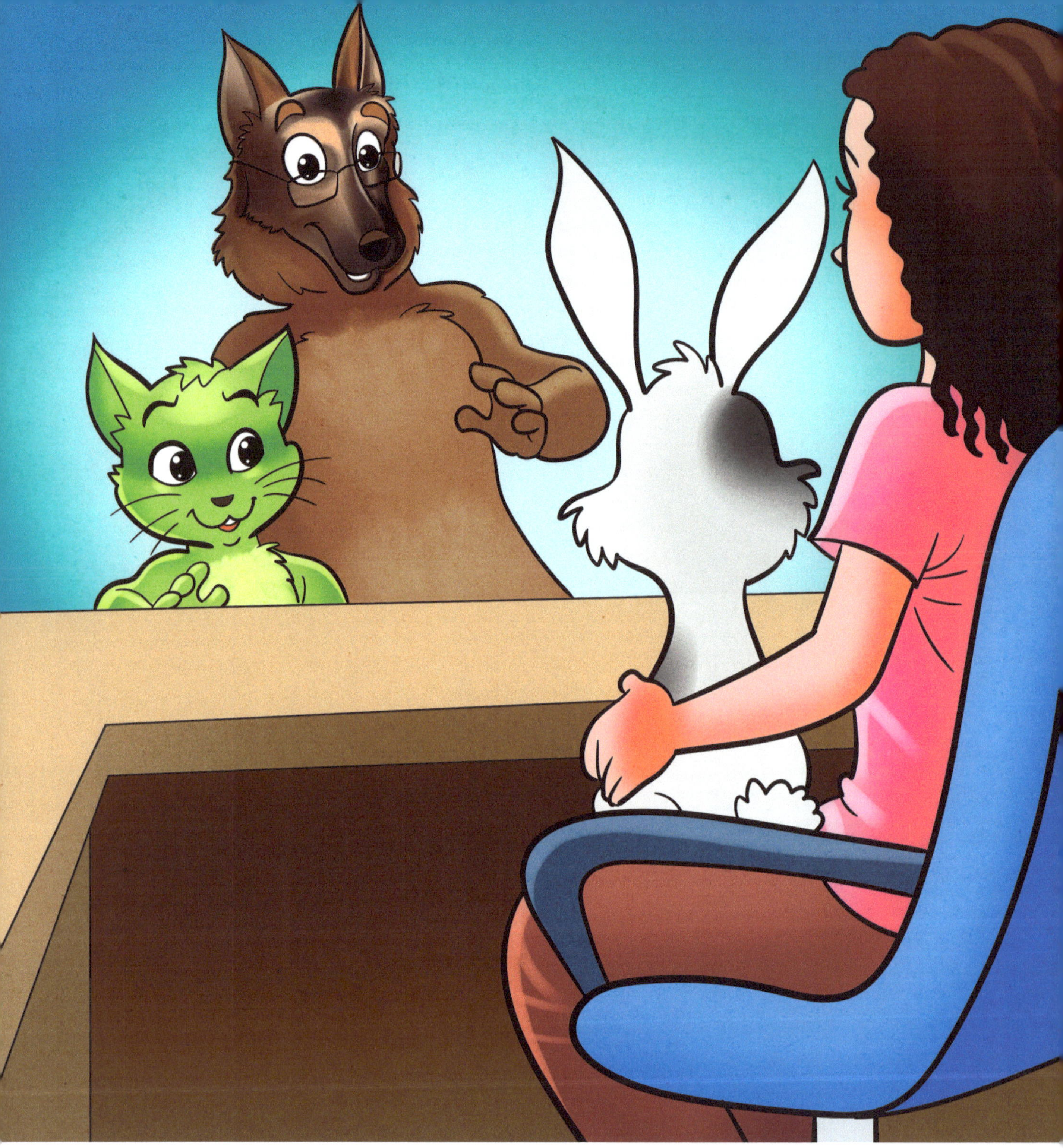

At that moment, Marlon Bundo's giant ears appear!
"Yes!" says Cannabis.
"Marlon, we were all worried about you!" says Major.
Marlon jumps up and says, "I've decided I'm not moving back to Indiana!"

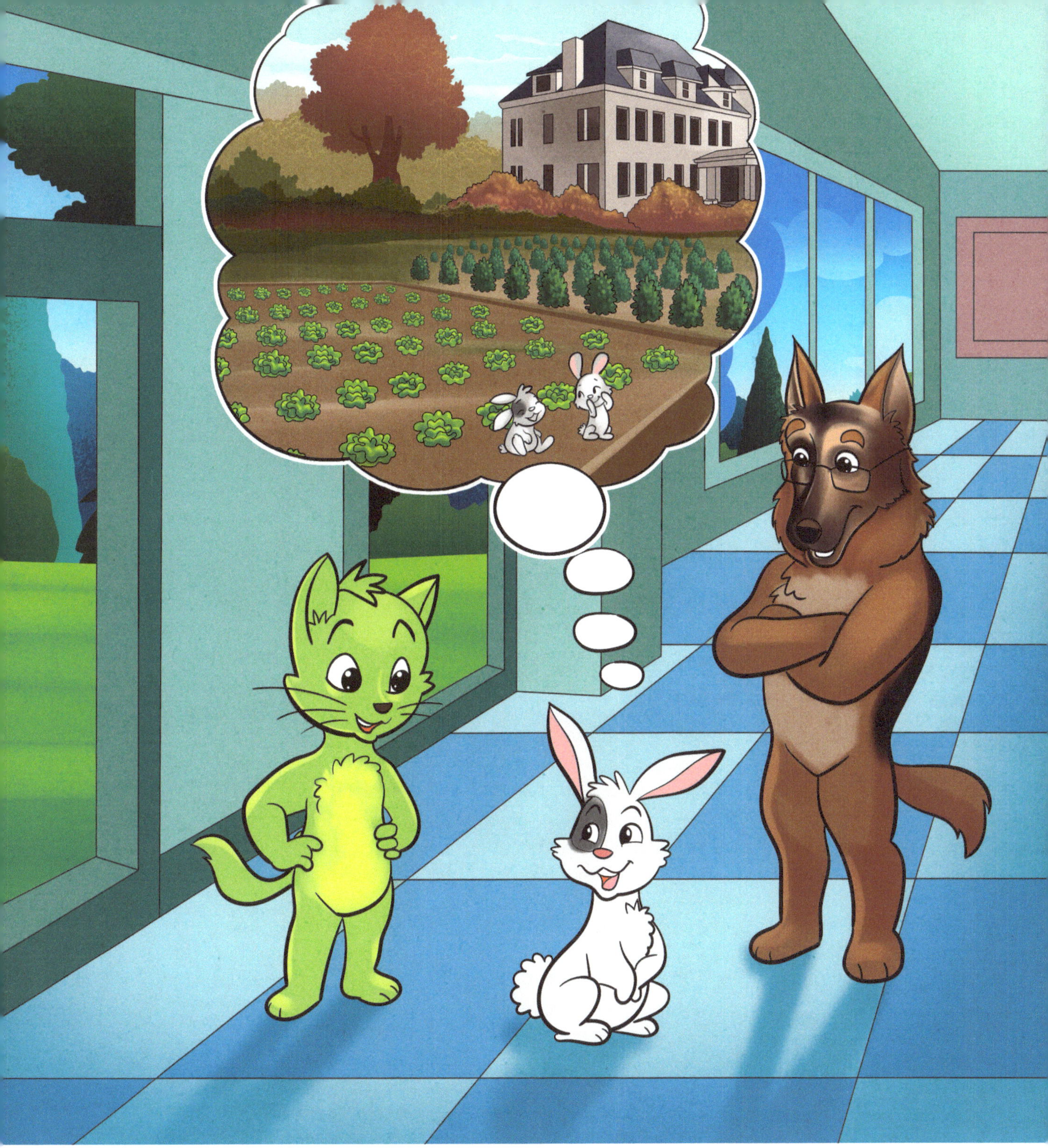

Once Marlon learned that Arthur was at the Vice President's vegetable garden, Marlon knew exactly where he wanted to live. And the three of them flew off to the Naval One Observatory to tell Arthur the great news!

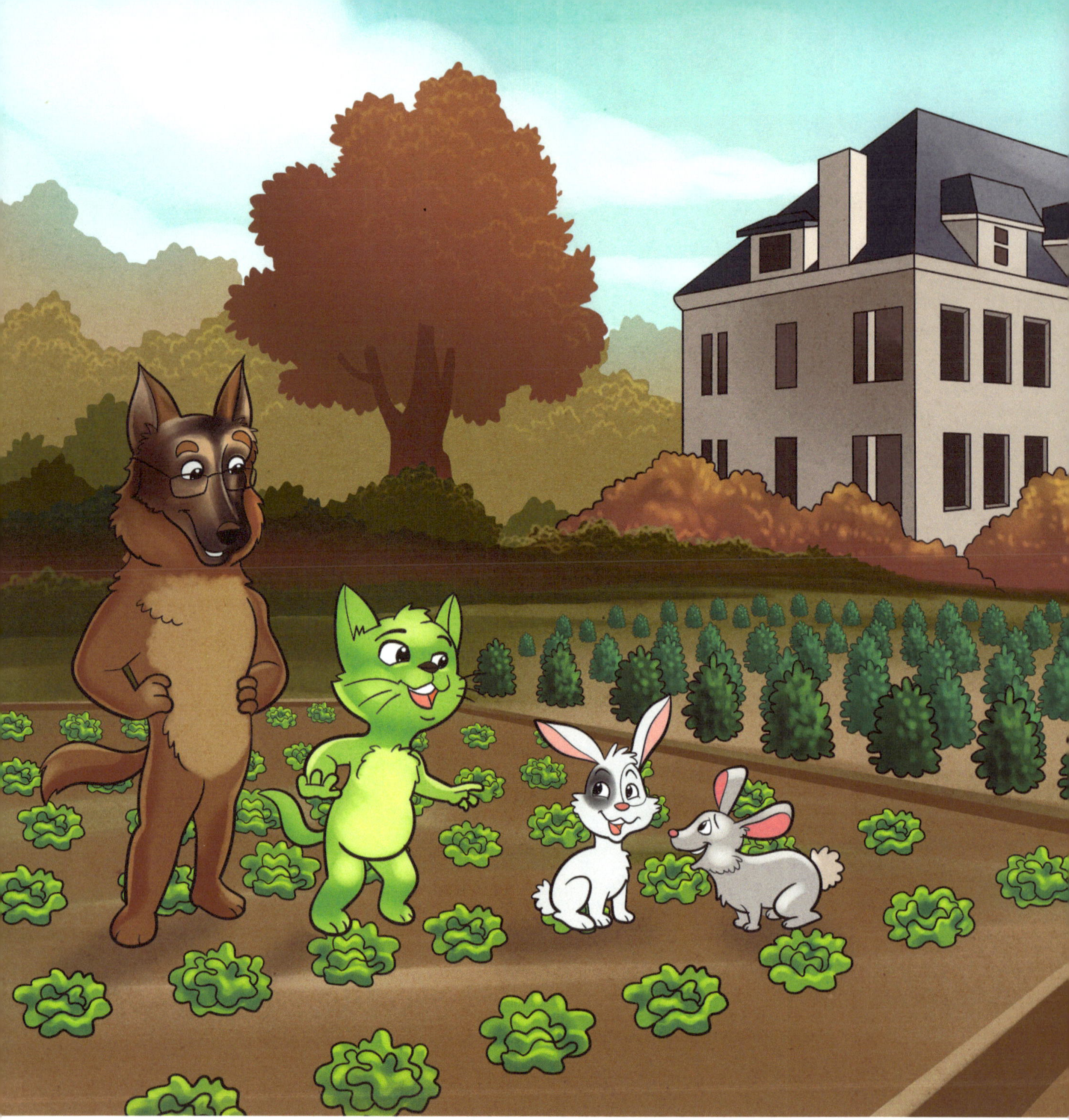

"Hurray! It's my friend Marlon Bundo. I was so worried about you. Are you okay?" asks Arthur.

"Yes, I'm okay," says Marlon. "I'm sorry for making you worry. I've decided I'm staying in DC. I want my birthday cake, and I wanna eat it too!" They both smiled and laughed together.

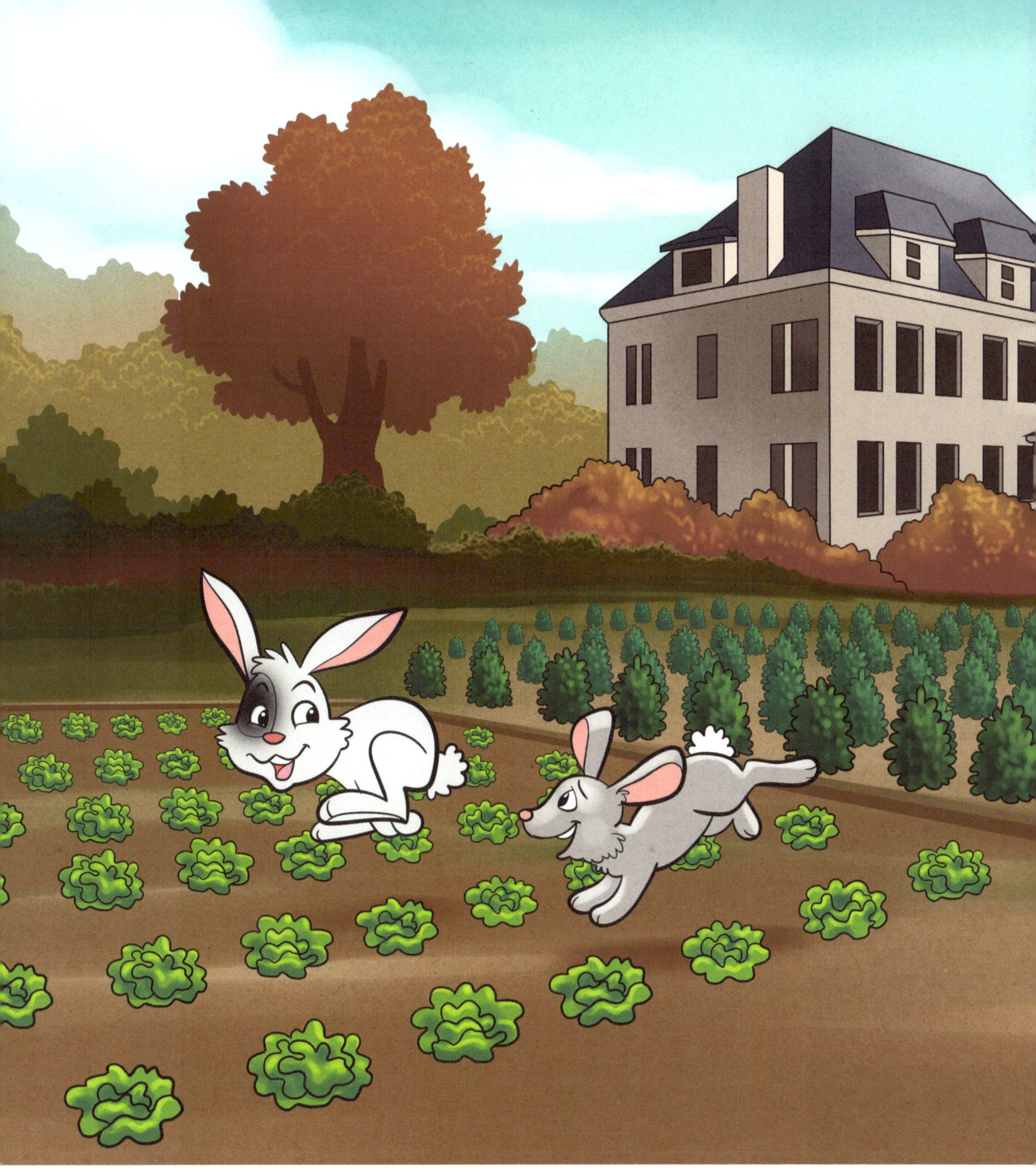

So bunny rabbits Arthur and Marlon lived happily ever after in the vegetable garden of Kamala Harris, our country's first black woman to become Vice President of the United States.

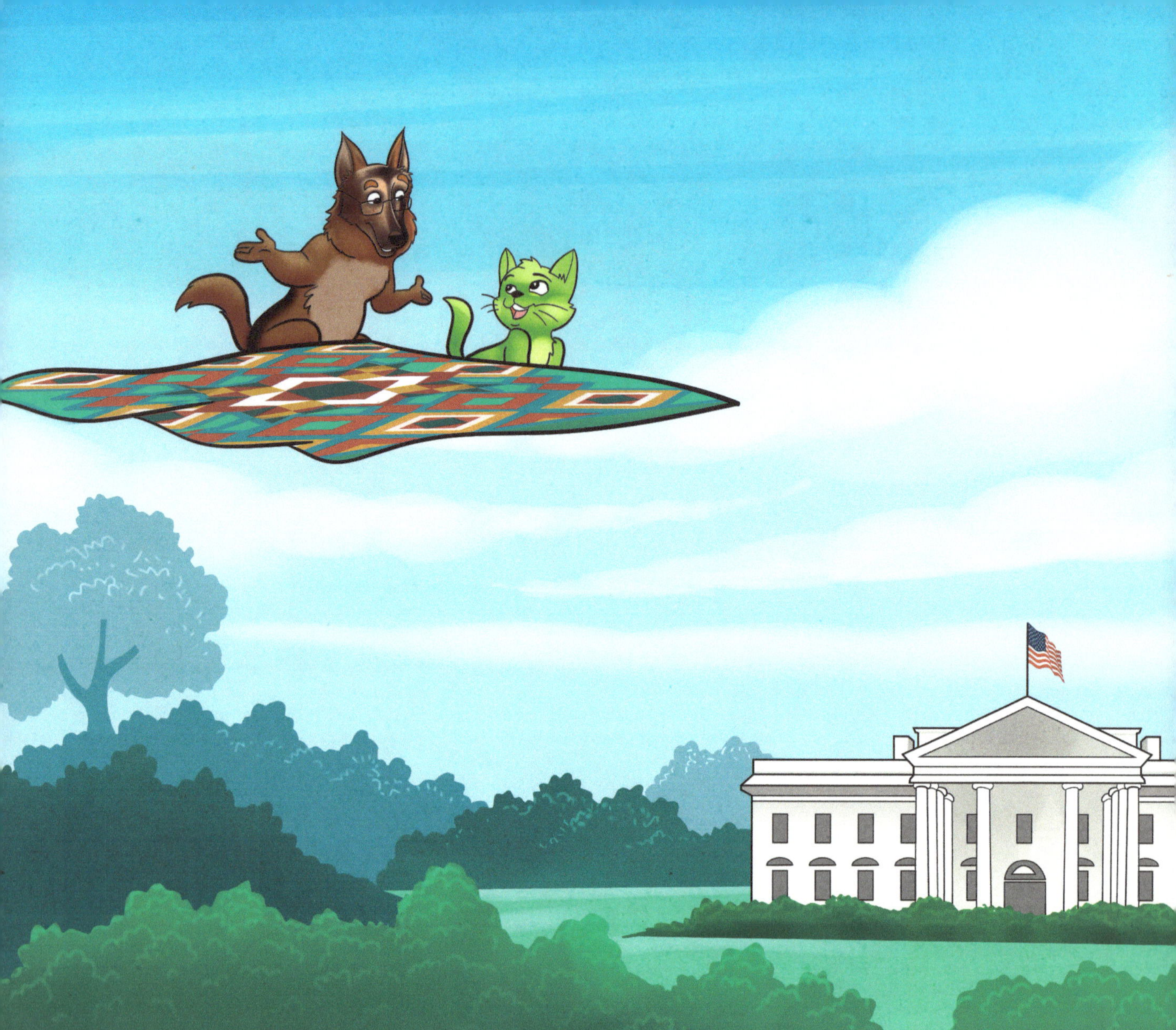

"Cannabis, can you take me home to the White House?" asks Major.

"I sure can," says Cannabis.

"Joe should be getting home soon, and I can't wait to tell him that you don't have to use marijuana to love Cannabis The Cat!" The two laughed out loud.

Then Cannabis says, "And I'll always remember to visit the Humane Society when looking for a friend. And Cannabis the Cat and Major fly off for the White House.

The End

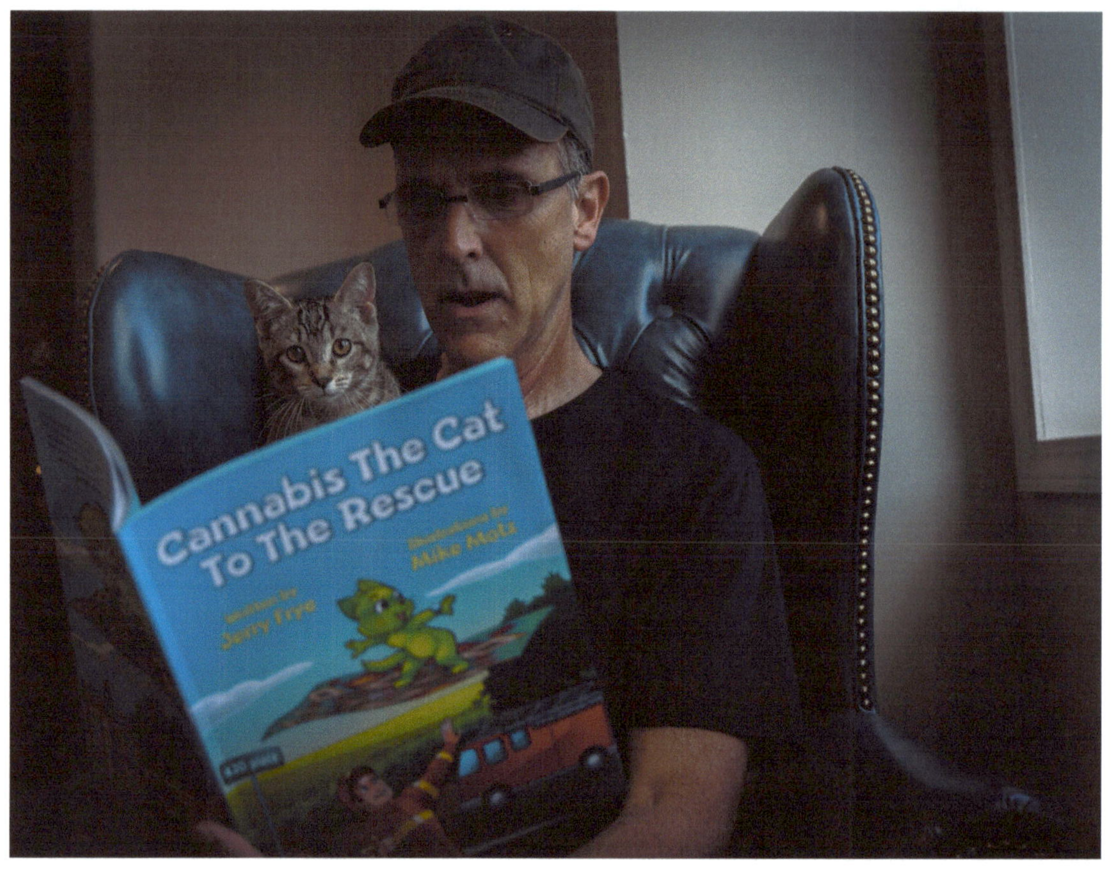

Meet Jerry Frye

Jerry Frye is a Navy veteran, former firefighter, and father of three. After years of battling alcoholism, he was able to finally stop drinking. At age 50 he earned a college degree with an emphasis in addiction studies. Today he celebrates 14 years without alcohol, enjoys traveling, investing in real estate, and lives with his cat named Cannabis.